# WOMEN HEALERS

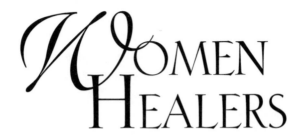

# WOMEN HEALERS

## PORTRAITS OF HERBALISTS, PHYSICIANS, AND MIDWIVES

### ELISABETH BROOKE

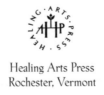

Healing Arts Press
Rochester, Vermont

Healing Arts Press
One Park Street
Rochester, Vermont 05767

*Note to the reader: This book is intended as an informational guide. The remedies, approaches, and techniques described herein are meant to supplement, and not to be a substitute for, professional medical care or treatment. They should not be used to treat a serious ailment without prior consultation with a qualified healthcare professional.*

LIBRARY OF CONGRESS CATALOGING-IN-PUBLICATION DATA

Brooke, Elisabeth.
    Women healers : portraits of herbalists, physicians, and midwives /
Elisabeth Brooke.
        p.        cm.
    "Originally published in Great Britain by the Women's Press Ltd. in 1993"
—T.p. verso.
    Includes bibliographical references and index.
    ISBN 0-89281-548-5
    1. Women healers.   2. Women in medicine.   I. Title.   II Title:
Women healers through history
R692.B76   1995
610.69'082—dc20                                                            95-23433
                                                                                    CIP
Printed and bound in the United States

10  9  8  7  6  5  4  3  2  1

Text design and layout by Kris Camp
This book was typeset in Minion, with Phaistos and Shelley as display typefaces.

Healing Arts Press is a division of Inner Traditions International

Distributed to the book trade in Canada by Publishers Group West (PGW), Toronto, Ontario
Distributed to the health food trade in Canada by Alive Books, Toronto and Vancouver

THE AUTHOR WOULD LIKE TO THANK THE FOLLOWING:
    The *British Medical Journal*, for quotations from "The media on the Cleveland Affair," by Harvey Marcovitch, 16 July 1988.
    Cambridge University Press, for quotations from *Women Writers of the Middle Ages* by Peter Dronke, 1984, and *Women as Healers: A History of Women and Medicine* by Hillary Bourdillon, 1988.
    The *Lancet*, for quotations from "Professional implications of the Savage Case," 12 April 1986.
    Oxford University Press, for quotations from *Medieval Women's Visionary Literature* by E. Petroff, 1986.
    University of Oklahoma Press, for quotations from *Medicine Women, Curanderas, and Women Doctors,* by Bobette Perrone, H. Henrietta Stockel, and Victoria Krueger. Copyright 1989 by Bobette Perrone, H. Henrietta Stockel, and Victoria Krueger. Published by the University of Oklahoma Press.
    Virago Press, for quotations from *A Savage Enquiry: Who Controls Childbirth?* by Wendy Savage, 1986.
    The Women's Press Ltd, for quotations from *The Charge of the Parasols* by Catriona Blake, first published 1990, and *Women and Nature* by Susan Griffin, first published in Great Britain, 1984.
    Every effort has been made to trace the original copyright holders, but in some instances this has not been possible. It is hoped that any such omission from this list will be excused.

# Contents

*In memoriam*

Manuel Luis Cherisme. "Papó."
September 1962–May 1992

Infinito

> El silencio escucha la muerte
> que se acerca,
> enciende  las luces y espera,
> mucho sabe esperar;
> puede ir y venir
> pero; espera,
> el es el tiempo mismo

Duluc
Santo Domingo

# $\mathscr{A}$cknowledgments

THIS BOOK WAS WRITTEN UNDER the most difficult circumstances and finished under tragic ones. Acknowledgments should be a happy recognition of the support a writer has found in the writing of her book. These acknowledgments bear witness to a deeper kind of support, in response to a tragedy in my life.

The writing of the book was done in my Caribbean home, with my new family from Mata de los Indios in Villa Mella and in La Ceja in La Romana. At times the surreal nature of writing about European history in the Caribbean struck me forcibly, and at others it made complete sense in the context of the lives of the two communities who adopted me. Women's struggles remain the same whatever the class, race, or century. The fight against bigotry remains as sharp as ever, and women and men still die for challenging the status quo.

The women of the community of Mata de los Indios supported me in the writing of this book through their care and friendship and their constant reminders not to worry so much, to work too hard, and take myself too seriously. Especial thanks go to my dear friend, Ibelisi Brazoban, and her mother, Selo Brazoban. Diana Rosario gave me her loving friendship, and her faith in my work brought me through difficult times. Duluc beguiled me with his song and poetry and encouraged the artist in me. Annie McMorris kindly let me type the manuscript on her computer, and Cecilia and Patricia from the Catholic Institute of International Relations gave me use of their office when the Santo Domingo electricity corporation presented us with eighteen-hour power cuts.

That this book has emerged at all is due, in great part, to my editor and friend, Loulou Brown. While I could hardly put one foot in front of the other, she and I painstakingly edited the manuscript. Her patience and care sustained me in what were some of the very darkest times. Her hard work has ironed out the confusions and curtailed my ramblings.

I would also like to thank the women from The Women's Press, especially Kathy Gale and Liz Gibbs, for their compassion and thoughtfulness. And my agent, Jane Judd, who protected me from the worst vicissitudes of publishing and whose support has kept me going. I would like to thank the staff of the Wellcome Institute for the History of Medicine Library, the British Library, and the Marylebone Medical Library for their help in researching this book.

And finally, I would like to thank the women in my life into whose arms I fell, and who, as always, sustained and healed me—Vita Revelli, Maggie Hyde, Maxine Holden, Mary Swale, and Helen Stapelton; and also my brother, Christopher Brooke, for his friendship. Thank you all.

Elisabeth Brooke
London, Lammas 1992

# $\mathcal{I}$ntroduction

MEDICINE IS DEEPLY POLITICAL AND HAS ALWAYS BEEN SO. The priestess-healers of ancient times wielded tremendous power as does the medical hierarchy today. The form taken by the prevailing politics determines who will be the physicians and who the patients. Will only the rich, whites, and Christians have access to health care? The reader will see that, with a few notable exceptions, the politics of Europe have been defined by white, male, Christian values. That is they have been, and are, racist, sexist, homophobic, and anti-Semitic. The struggle to prevent the "underclasses" from practicing medicine has been constant and bloody. The ruling class has naturally endeavored to keep tight control over the professions and scholarship, so history also reflects this patriarchal and racist bias. Women, however, have now begun their own historical studies and are reconstructing history to reflect the experience of the majority of the world's population.

The sources for this book are few and far between, and therefore the accounts of the women's lives portrayed are at times infuriatingly sketchy. Lack of resources and publishing constraints mean that black women hardly feature in this book—except for the discussion of ancient Egypt in chapter 1 and the redoubtable Mary Seacole in chapter 8. No work of feminist scholarship is complete without the voices of black women, and I trust black women and other women of color will continue this work.

Before I began, I had no idea that women had been doctors for thousands of years, let alone that before patriarchal times they were considered to be the natural healers. I had been led to believe it was our battling Victorian great-grandmothers who were the first doctors. I hope my book will show this is far from the case.

Women have always been healers. This book is a brief journey through the lives of our healing foremothers. From myth and poetry to the well-documented Victorian campaigners, we see women fighting and sometimes dying for the right to practice medicine. This book is a study and a celebration of the brave, inspired, and, above all, determined women healers of the past. I have gathered together the fragments of their lives and work that have remained safe from historical censors. Where women have been portrayed in medicine, they are seen as ministering angels (which many were) but in an ancillary and unpaid, hence "unprofessional" capacity. If they remained faithful to their class and prevailing patriarchal value systems, they were remembered. Hence, we know of Florence Nightingale but nothing of Mary Seacole; Elizabeth Garrett-Anderson had a hospital named after her, whereas Sophia Jex-Blake has for the most part long been forgotten.

Some women were surgeons, some general practitioners, some obstetricians, and others professors of medicine. Their lives, except for contemporary women, have not been recorded in great detail.

I have resisted the temptation to speculate about their practice, so at times the information is sparse. But I felt it was preferable to include whatever brief account of their lives I could find.

One familiar picture of the woman healer is that of the wise woman, the witch-healer who lived and still lives in rural areas throughout the world. She is the primary health care worker for most of the world's population who do not have access to modern medicine. The average reader may conjure up a picture of the witch of medieval times who, by means of spells, charms, and incantations, healed the sick, made barren women fertile, bewitched cattle, and the like—and who, if she fell foul of the local lord, would end up on the ducking stool or be roasted at the stake. Women healers have been represented as quaint, unsavory, harmless, or wicked, depending on the point of view. I hope my book will show this is in fact far from the case and that attacks on "mad old women" who were called witches were in reality an orchestrated campaign to wipe out any opposition to the rule of the church. Woman-hating dogma is an integral part of Christianity, and the church's avowed intent is the preservation of white, male domination.

There is another history of the woman healer. She was an innovative, scientific, humane, and caring practitioner. She worked alongside her male colleagues and shared her insights and discoveries with them, often to find them stolen or not accredited to her. She built hospitals, taught in medical schools, developed theories, pioneered new methods of treatment, and discoursed with the great thinkers of her time. Yet she often practiced under threat of death. Why was it that women in medicine were so discriminated against? To answer this question, we need to go back to cultures in which it was accepted that women should practice medicine, to a time when female goddesses were worshiped and the Great Mother ruled supreme.

The worship of the Great Mother, as practiced in ancient Egypt, Greece, and Rome, was generally centered around moon worship. The three phases of the moon were seen to represent the three faces of woman: maiden, mother, and crone. The priestess-healer and the sibyl or prophetess personified the goddess as virgin. Virgin in the sense she was owned by no man, the priestess-healer would interpret omens and answer questions about sickness through the use of trance, dreams, astrology, tarot, and runes. Healing rituals would be performed within the temples as prescribed by the goddess. The full moon related to mother figures who worked with childbirth and practiced general medicine, which women like Trotula and Hildegard personified. The dark of the moon shows the crone face of the goddess. She is Hecate, dweller in the shadows, who deals with death and madness. She communicates with spirits of the netherworlds and may be a shaman.

The ancient world knew the Great Mother and yet chose to forget her. Upstart gods appeared until she was finally unseated by Jehovah, the wrathful, avenging god. He showed her no mercy and cut her down. His followers mirrored his matricide, and women, once revered, were raped, murdered, and enslaved. Captive and powerless, they found that no area of public life was open to them, and one by one, their rights were removed while their areas of influence diminished. Women physicians were outlawed and forbidden to practice medicine. Men resented the respect and power practicing medicine had given them. Over the years women have been tolerated as physicians where the power of the church was least. Trotula, for example, came from a part of Italy renowned for its pagan practices. Hildegard, of course, could not be called a pagan, but she had the good fortune to be a highly intelligent mystic and was safe from the worst excesses of the inquisitors.

As the Middle Ages were succeeded by the Renaissance, repression became more bloody and culminated in the wholesale slaughter of millions of women, many of whom were herbalists, midwives, mystics, and nurses. Gradually, women started using the law to make their case to practice as licensed doctors alongside men. Women of the nineteenth century fought a legal, but in the end no less bloody, battle to be treated on an equal footing with male practitioners. One of men's main fears was that women would outshine them in their degree courses, which they proceeded to do. Finally they won through, though women in medicine are still having to defend their right to practice.

There is a growing revulsion against male-dominated, mechanistic medicine. Medical ethics are constantly debated in a mad world where the old and terminally ill cannot elect to die in peace and the brain-dead are kept alive by machines. Unfashionable areas of medicine, such as mental health, are starved of the resources, both human and financial, that could effect real change.

In the minefield that is medicine, women's voices are urgently needed to bring some common sense into the debate. What use is nuclear medicine or operations on fetuses while much of the world suffers and dies from easily preventable diseases?

Whether we work in conventional or alternative medicine, the fact that we are women healers gives us common ground. The political issues apply to both fields. It is naive to imagine that alternative medicine is any less sexist or racist than conventional medicine. Women health workers will understand more about the complex issues involved in their practice, and women patients will likewise be able to make clearer choices about their treatment if both can appreciate the way women have suffered throughout history, particularly in medicine.

Women doctors, therapists, nurses, midwives, and alternative medicine practitioners are all urgently needed to voice their opposition to the medical orthodoxy that has changed the life-giving art of healing into the deadly science of modern medicine. I hope this book will help to implement the changes needed.

# 1

# $\mathcal{H}$ealing in Antiquity

## ANCIENT EGYPT

Ancient Egypt had a highly organized and greatly respected healing tradition which merged the roles of priest or priestess and physician. The sicknesses of the body and of the soul were seen to be connected, if not intimately linked. Most healers worked with healing goddesses, using a combination of spiritual practice and practical medical techniques. Medicine was a highly sophisticated art in ancient Egypt, far in advance of many of the nearby cultures. Physicians took charge of mummifying the dead and performing ritual circumcision, and female obstetricians took care of women in labor, bringing them to the birth houses in the temples of Isis. They would use astrology to predict how the birth would proceed and what problems might occur. During labor, while the temple midwives attended the woman, she would sit on warmed stones and be given healing massages to ease the pain of contractions and to relax the uterus.

### Isis

Isis was the major healing goddess of the Egyptians. She was known as the restorer of life and the source of healing herbs. She was identified with the healing star Sirius, which forms part of the constellation of

Canis Major. This star appears on the horizon just as the Nile begins to flood and was thus seen by the Egyptians as the harbinger of fertility and abundance. It was Isis who dispensed healing herbs and protected women in childbirth. She could restore sight to the blind and sensibility to a paralyzed leg or arm. She gave strength to those who had been weakened by illness, and she would visit the sick as they lay in bed. Her wings would brush across their bodies, cleansing and healing them, and she would give voice to healing chants and incantations.

Priestesses of Isis were always dressed in white, the favorite color of the goddess. The altars of her numerous temples would be decorated with white flowers, berries, and vervain, the plant sacred to her. A wax model of the sick person would be placed on the altar. The healing rituals were long and complicated. The incantations had to be sung in a particular way; otherwise, they would have no effect. The patient would bring offerings of food and clothes. Talismans would be prepared, and healing massages were given, while the patient consumed herbal drinks.

Egypt was a center for healing temples, and people came from far away to be healed. Many sacred places were situated in health resorts and in major cities throughout the kingdom, some of the most popular of which were the temples of Isis. Others, at Heliopolis and Saïs, were later expanded into medical schools. Sais specialized in gynecology and obstetrics.

A tablet found there reads: "I have come from the school of medicine at Heliopolis, and have studied at the woman's school at Saïs where the divine mothers have taught me how to cure diseases."[1]

The Ebers papyrus, which has been dated to around 1550 B.C.E., contains hundreds of recipes, including some for women's diseases. Believed to have been written for the medical students at Saïs, the following invocation is to be found at its beginning:

> As it is to be, a thousand times. This is the book for the healing of all diseases. May Isis heal me even as she healed Horus of all the pains which his brother Set had inflicted on him when he killed his brother Osiris! O Isis, thou great enchantress, heal me, deliver me from all evil, bad typhonic things, from demoniacal

and deadly diseases and pollutions of all sorts that rush upon
me, as thou didst deliver and release thy son Horus.[2]

On the walls in the Hall of Rolls in Heliopolis are inscriptions and
votive tablets. A list of diseases and cures was kept with the medical
papyri, which the priestess-healers would have looked after. Charms
and prayers would be recited. The temples were highly organized
places, and the practice of medicine was divided so that a physician
worked only in his or her specialty of medicine. Herodotus said:
"All the country is full of physicians, some of the eye, some of the
teeth, some of what pertains to the belly, and some of the hidden
disease."[3]

Several medical papyri that show the depth and extent of Egyptian
medical practice have been found.[4] The Kahun papyrus, dated around
1900 B.C.E., covers the diseases of women and children. As only women
treated women's ailments, this text was written for women practitioners. It contains formulas for deciding whether a woman was barren
or fertile. Sterility was treated with animal glands, an ancient precursor
of synthetic hormone treatments. The following remedy was for a
prolapsed uterus:

> Examination of a woman whose back aches, and the inside of her
> thighs are painful. Say to her it is the falling of the womb. Do
> thus for her: ua grains, shasha fruit 5 ro [1 ro = 1 teaspoon],
> cow's milk 1 hnw [1 pint], cook, let it cool, make it into a gruel,
> and drink for four "mornings".[5]

To promote conception it was suggested that a woman mix incense,
fresh fat dates, and sweet beer and burn the mixture on a fire.

The priestess-healers were also responsible for cultivating the medicinal herb gardens and oversaw the preparation of remedies in the
pharmacies. The oldest pictorial representation of a female physician
has been dated to around 3000 B.C.E. It shows Isis with a male child
who has a withered, paralyzed leg. He was brought before the goddess
who healed him.[6]

Records have been found of a woman physician who practiced in the reign of Queen Neferirika-ra, around 2730 B.C.E. She is believed to have been one of the healers working at Saïs.

The female dynasty of Egyptian queens, which began around 4000 B.C.E., promoted and encouraged medical and scientific practice. The queens themselves were almost always physicians, and some were renowned as skilled practitioners.

## Hatshepsut

Queen Hatshepsut reigned from 1503 to 1482 B.C.E. She promoted and encouraged women practitioners. She was known as a wise and benevolent queen, and her reign has been called the golden age of Egyptian culture. Hatshepsut's deeds are only now being rediscovered after very many centuries. Her jealous brothers, who erased eulogies to her, pretended her great works were theirs. She was both a pacifist and a philosopher. In the temple of Hathor, the birth of the queen is shown, with the ram and frog gods in attendance imploring aid from the ibis god. Hatshepsut was given milk by Hathor, who was her protectress.

Hatshepsut encouraged all her subjects to study. She started up three medical schools, as well as founding botanical and herb gardens for the propagation of medicinal plants.

Gradually, as the female dynasty came to an end, the role of women healers diminished, and male priests and healers took over the practice of medicine. The medical schools continued to flourish, however, and were the training ground for many of the classical Greek physicians.

## ANCIENT GREECE

Some of the oldest surgical techniques come from ancient Greece where medicine incorporated the use of herbs, massage, and incantations to healing goddesses. Healing charms were used, together with prayers in rituals for the sick and dying. Surgery was used only as a last resort but was practiced to a high standard. It may well have been women who were responsible for the development of surgical techniques and therapeutics, especially in the disciplines of physiology, anatomy, obstetrics, and pathology.

Evidence for women healers can be found in ancient Greek litera-ture. For example, in the *Iliad* there is a reference to Agamede, the daughter of Angea, the king of the Epei, who cared for the wounded and dying Greeks lying on the battlefields of Troy. She was:

> *Agamede, with golden hair*
> *A leech was she, and well she knew all herbs on*
> *ground that grew.*
> *She washed the gory wounds of the dying Trojans, giving*
> *them cordial drinks and "the gentle bath."*[7]

In the *Odyssey*, a leech known as Polydamna, whose name signifies the one who subdues diseases, is mentioned. Polydamna gave Helen of Troy the famous nepenthe to poison her enemies or cure her friends. She was supposed to have lived at Thebes between 2000 and 1780 B.C.E. Nepenthe was variously claimed to have been elecampane, verbena (the remedy of Isis), poppy, or evening primrose.[8]

## Gaia

The shrine at Delphi was sacred to Gaia, the earth goddess, and medi-cal treatment there was similar to a twilight sleep (i.e., a trance-like state to induce auto-suggestive ideas akin to hypnosis). Medicinal plants were used as well as massage, medicinal baths, purges, bleedings, water from sacred springs, and forms of exercise. The seer, called Pythia, sat on a stool around which was wrapped a python. Her utterances were not often intelligible, so the priestesses had to translate the words that came from the oracle. The shrine was taken over by the patriarchal god Apollo, who killed the python. Drawings and sculptures reveal that these women priestesses were guarded by the Amazon warriors. There are scenes showing them fighting with male invaders who defeated them, sad to say, and took over this most holy of healing shrines.[9]

## Panacea and Hygeia

Aesculapius and his healing family were believed to have lived around 900 B.C.E. in Greece. Over 300 temples and sanatoriums were built to him and his two daughters, Panacea, who was invoked to restore good health and to conserve it, and Hygeia, the goddess of health and conserver of good health, and to his wife Epione, who was the patron saint of those in pain. In the healing space or *abaton* in the temples the patients were drugged or hypnotized into altered states of consciousness. The gods and goddesses would then appear to them and give them healing. Snakes figured strongly in the healing arts and were used in divination. Their venom is believed to have been used to induce a dreamless sleep in the patients. In the ritual for treatment, the patients were taken into the bathhouses for ablutions and then brought to feed the sacred snakes. Subsequently they gave cakes to the dogs, paid the priestesses, and then lay on the marble beds to dream.

## Agnodice

Agnodice, an Athenian woman, is credited with starting the female medical revolution that began in Athens and later spilled over into the whole of the Greek empire. The ancient Roman author Hyginus wrote about her.[10] Agnodice had wanted to study medicine, but at the time medical study and practice were forbidden to women on pain of death. She decided to disguise herself as a man and went to study with one of the most famous physicians, Herophilos, at the medical school in Alexandria. She felt called to practice and was prepared to risk the death penalty to exercise what she felt to be her natural right. She was driven to become a doctor because so many women were dying unnecessarily in Athens as they refused to be treated by male physicians. She was outraged by this and was determined to do whatever she could to remedy the situation.

When she finished her studies, she set up a practice in Athens, again disguised as a man. Once the local women discovered her secret, they flocked to her door. She was found out by jealous male colleagues, who denounced her to the courts. She was arrested and brought before the judge. Tried and found guilty of the illegal practice of medicine, she was sentenced to death. When her women patients heard of this, they marched on the courthouse. They threatened to commit mass suicide if Agnodice were not set free and the sentence dismissed. The judges had no choice but to acquiesce, as many of their wives and daughters were among the wealthy women demanding justice. From this time onward, all gentlewomen (that is, those who were not slaves and foreigners) were permitted to study and practice medicine. Though they were only permitted to treat women and children, the financial rewards were great, and this gave the women physicians economic independence as well as a freedom unknown to other Greek women.

## Theano

Theano was the wife of Pythagoras, the philosopher mathematician, who studied and practiced medicine. When he died, she took over the running of his school, teaching philosophy and medicine. She was famous for her knowledge of medical science and philosophy of medicine.

## Pythias

Pythias was the wife of Aristotle (384–322 B.C.E.). She made a special study of botany, biology, and embryology. She owned a vast collection of manuscripts and was coauthor of many of her husband's works—although he calls her his "assistant." She honeymooned on the island of Mytilone, made famous by Sappho, the lesbian poet.

## Artemisia

Artemisia was the queen of Caria (d. 355 B.C.E.). She was a great and famous healer who had a wide knowledge of medicinal plants. According to Pliny, she was credited with discovering the value of the plant wormwood as a drink, which was named after her: Artemisia.[11]

## Aspasia

Aspasia, another famous Greek woman physician, practiced in Rome as well as in Athens. A fresco over the portal of the main building at the university of Athens shows her in the company of such august figures as Socrates, Plato, Archimedes, and Sophocles. She practiced in the first century C.E. Fragments of her writing remain today, quoted in the *Telrabilion* of Aetius (527–566 C.E.), which was printed in 1534. Her work remained the standard gynecological text until the time of Trotula.

Aspasia specialized in gynecology and obstetrics. She described the many fetal positions and researched ways to prevent miscarriages. She recommended diets and exercise for pregnant women to reduce their labor pains. During a difficult labor, she recommended dilating the cervix by applying hot lotions (for instance, olive oil, mallow, flax seed) to the vulva. For pushing out a retained placenta, she recommended the woman close her mouth and nose and attempt to breathe out. She devised various contraceptives using tampons soaked in herbal preparations such as oak gall, myrrh, and wine. These are well-known astringent remedies that dry up the vaginal secretions, thus hindering the movement of sperm up the vagina. In the case of a retroverted or anteverted uterus, she believed the cause was congestion of the liver veins, which would affect the bowels, engorging them and putting pressure on the uterus. Her treatment entailed using pessaries (tar, bitumen, and hot oil) and replacing the uterus with the fingers. Aspasia also described how she performed operations to remove uterine tumors and to treat peritonitis. In her treatment of fibroids of the uterus, she operated to remove them and then inserted tampons soaked in red earth, rose water, mandragora, and hemlock. She also described the surgical procedures for hernia and varicose veins.

## Antiochis

A physician named Antiochis had a statue erected to her by her grateful patients in the town of Tlos. The inscription reads: "Antiochis, daughter of Diodotos of Tlos the council and the commune of the city of Tlos in appreciation of her medical ability, erected at their own expense this statue in her honour."[12]

In his *De Compositione Medicamentorum Liber*, Galen, writing in the second century C.E., acknowledged the writings of many medical women, including Antiochis's prescriptions for chest pain and gout.

## Cleopatra

Cleopatra was a physician practicing at the time of Galen (129–201 C.E.). She wrote a vast work on gynecology, which was copied and circulated throughout the Greco-Roman world. It was used by physicians and midwives until well into the sixteenth century as a standard medical reference work. Parts were published in 1566 in *Harmonia Gynaecorum* by Wolff and Spach. It is believed she may have been Arsinoe's sister. Cleopatra has been confused with several other women of the same name, including the queen, who knew about poisons, and other healers who lived at the time of Galen. Only when it was printed, many centuries after she had died, was her work once again attributed to her. Her works are believed to have been extensively plagiarized by Soranus who reproduced many of them in his opus *Gynaecology*, which became a standard text for several hundred years.

# ANCIENT ROME

Increasing numbers of Greek physicians, famous for their medical skill and expertise, came to practice in Rome around 200 B.C.E. Women, then allowed to practice as physicians, came with the male practitioners. They treated Roman women, who were delighted to have women healers attending them. Women physicians were much sought after and were able to command high fees. Among these successful practitioners were Victoria and Leoparda, both mentioned by the medical writer Theodorus Priscianus. He dedicated the third book of *Rerum Medicarum* to Victoria, and in his preface speaks of her as not only a practitioner with an accurate knowledge of medicine but also as one who was a keen observer and experienced physician.

Monuments and inscriptions on tombstones reveal that Roman *medicae* (women doctors) practiced not only obstetrics and midwifery but also general medicine. A funeral tablet found in Portugal tells of a woman who was a most excellent physician *(medica optima)*, while another describes the deceased as mistress of medical science *(antistes disciplinae in medicina fuit)*.[13] Prior to 100 C.E. women were allowed into the professions but needed to be circumspect. Celsus described women doctors in Rome, together with their slaves, examining urine, applying leeches, and administering poppy juice as an anesthetic for surgery.[14]

## Olympias

In 50 C.E. Pliny described Olympias, a woman in Thebes, who wrote a valuable book on prescriptions. It contained a chapter on the diseases of women, another on preventing abortion, and one on causing an abortion if this was deemed necessary.[15]

## Octavia

Many women physicians were from aristocratic families. For instance, Octavia, the first wife of Mark Anthony, wrote a book of prescriptions. For toothache, she recommended barley, honey, flour, vinegar, and salt, which were all to be baked, pulverised with charcoal, and scented with flowers. Her remedies were described by Scibonius Largus, physician to the Emperor Claudius, in the first century C.E.[16]

## St. Theodosia

Christianity gradually became the dominant religion throughout the Roman Empire. Christian women took up the practice of medicine. Following Christ's teachings, many worked with the destitute, the sick, and the dying. Their names are legion, and several, such as St. Theodosia, were made into saints. She was the mother of the martyr St. Procopius and was distinguished for her knowledge of medicine and surgery, both of which she practiced in Rome with great success. She died by the sword during the persecution of Diocletian.

## St. Nicerata

St. Nicerata lived in Constantinople during the reign of the Emperor Aracadius. She is said to have cured St. John Chrysostom of an affliction of the stomach.

## Fabiola

Fabiola of Rome (d. 399 C.E.) converted to Christianity at age twenty and soon afterward married for the second time. When her second husband died soon after the marriage, she decided to devote herself to a life of charity. She was the daughter of one of the most illustrious patrician families in Rome. She studied medicine and became both physician and nurse. She opened a hospital in Ostia, which

> established a type of institution that was to effect more for ameliorating the condition of suffering humanity than anything that had before been dreamed of; something that was to contribute immensely to the efforts of physicians and surgeons in minimizing the sad ravages of wounds and disease.[17]

She also opened a hospital in Rome for the poor. The first of its kind, the hospital was soon inundated with the city's needy. This was an unheard-of innovation at the time and considered shocking by her contemporaries. Romans had little concept of charity and were quite uninterested in alleviating the suffering of the poor and needy. Fabiola became famous and was well loved by her fellow citizens, who were unused to acts of selflessness on the part of the Roman ruling classes. In 1854 Cardinal Wiseman said of her that "few physicians had so much moral or intellectual ability as she, so serious without pedantry, simple but not vulgar, quiet but deeply thoughtful."[18]

St. Jerome remarked that she was

> the glory of the church, the astonishment of the Gentiles, the mother of the poor and the consolation of the saints.... If I had a hundred tongues and a hundred mouths and iron lungs I should not be able to enumerate all the maladies to which Fabiola gave the most prodigal care and tenderness.[19]

When she died, thousands flocked to her funeral procession. It is said the streets of Rome were blocked for many hours.

# 2

# $\mathcal{M}$edicine in the Dark Ages

THE PERIOD FROM THE DECLINE OF THE ROMAN EMPIRE, around 300 C.E., until about the tenth century is known as the Dark Ages in Europe. During this time the continent was plunged into a darkness of spirit from which it was not to recover for hundreds of years.

Many reasons have been given for the long period of ignorance and baseness that followed the relatively advanced and enlightened Roman times. Although it is true the Romans were conquerors and patriarchs, nevertheless they encouraged the arts and learning of all kinds. They sponsored theater, dance, music, and encouraged scientific endeavor, as well as experiments in literature. But with the fall of Rome, ignorance, superstition, and crassness followed, and any form of sophistication or erudition in the Dark Ages was deemed to be suspect and condemned.

Barbara Walker[1] makes an interesting and original suggestion that the cause of this darkness was none other than Christianity. Christians actively and energetically opposed education and equated the spread of knowledge with the sign of the anti-Christ and the beginning of the end of the world. Once it became established, the church forbade education for laypeople, fearing that if people were educated they might well question the teachings of Christianity. One Christian put it thus: "those who know least of the principles of religion are the most earnest and fervent."[2]

Church leaders organized massive public book burnings and the destruction of libraries and schools. By the end of the fifth century, it was forbidden to study medicine, philosophy, mathematics, or geography. No Christian could study astronomy, while astrology was considered to be a diabolic art. All secular literature was denounced as wicked.

The church decreed that all schools of thought that deviated from its rigid and narrow viewpoint were heretical and devilish. The gospels that talked of God as mother and set out the contribution of women to the Christian movement and the teaching crusades of Jesus were excluded from the New Testament. This carefully contrived and calculated selection process, which was carried out by various Christian communities, was finished around the end of the second century. By that time almost all female representations of God and divinity had been erased. The censored works became known as the gnostic gospels[3] and included the gospels of Mary, Thomas, Philip, and the Secret Gospel of John. They depicted the feminine as both complementary and opposite to the masculine and as an integral part of God's creation, neither lesser nor greater than the masculine.

The church set about destroying all traces of pre-Christian culture and religious and philosophical thought, and it was almost completely successful. After years of wholesale and systematic destruction of books, parchments, scrolls, artworks, and music, little remained of the great civilizations of Europe and the Middle East. St. John Chrysostom boasted that "Every trace of the old philosophy and literature of the ancient world has vanished from the face of the earth."[4]

Pagan temples were systematically destroyed and churches and monasteries built on their sites. The Christians used materials from the demolished temples: gold, bronze, and silver artworks were melted down for money, and the marble gods and goddesses were broken down in lime kilns and used as mortar. In the fourth century Rome had 424 temples, but by the following century, these had all been destroyed. Eunapius, priest of the Eleusinian mysteries, described it as: "fabulous and formless darkness mastering the loveliness of the world."[5]

The church conducted a carefully calculated campaign to absorb and Christanize the more palatable parts of pagan beliefs. For example, important dates in the pagan calendar were taken over by the church. The pagan Samhain became All Saints' Day, while Yule became Christmas. Important pagan sites were invaded and churches built on them, Glastonbury being a significant example. Christian saints emerged to replace the pagan pantheon. For instance, Mary, mother of Jesus, replaced the fertile Queen of Heaven and became the impossible virgin mother, the pure asexual woman who conceived without intercourse with a man.

As the Christian influence grew, respect for the old ways waned, and society disintegrated and became corrupt. There was terrible inflation, crime, crippling taxes, and a general apathy and nihilistic attitude among ordinary people. Along with outbreaks of pestilence, famine, and epidemics, social standards fell, and moral codes degenerated sharply. While the rich bled the rest of the population, the poor rebelled by taking to the streets and looting and robbing others.

The advent of Christianity heralded a massive retrograde step for the whole of Western civilization. Education, generally, and the arts, culture, and any form of creative thinking were forbidden and suppressed. What had previously been a rich and diverse culture degenerated into a mass of superstition and ignorance.

All the professions suffered. The following quotation of Martial shows the popular opinion with regard to medicine in the century:

> A doctor once, Diaulos now
> Prepares men for the grave.
> A prudent man, he reaps the fruit
> Of all the drugs he gave.[6]

In the third century, there were great outbreaks of plague, famine, and unrest. Many educated people fled to Persia, Celtic Britain, and India to escape persecution. Sassan, King of Persia, started a great medical school and staffed it with many of the scholars who fled Europe. When Emperor Justinian closed the Greek schools, a wholesale exodus occurred.

The study of medicine was forbidden because the church taught that all diseases were caused by demons and could only be cured by the clergy exorcising them and using charms or holy relics. Any educated person was suspect, and ignorance was praised as this was said to engender piety as well as fear and admiration for those who could read and understand the Bible. Natural science and medicine suffered the most since experimentation or abstract thought could question Christian truths and express doubts. Thus, although it had been proved many centuries before that the earth was round, the church maintained that it was flat—and so flat it became. Anyone who believed otherwise was a heretic. It was taught, for example, that mice were generated asexually from decaying earth; that wasps emanated from the carcasses of dead horses and bees from dead calves; that a crab would turn into a scorpion if you cut off its legs; and that scorpions could be created from basil rubbed between two stones.[7]

Clearly, in this environment, no advance of science was possible. In fact scientific thought took several giant leaps backward. In the field of medicine, priestess-healers were an obvious target for the hostilities of the Christians. Not only were they heathen, they were wealthy and laid claim to a spiritual authority that directly threatened the church.

In the early days of Christianity, women were able to continue as healers and physicians, but as its patriarchal bias increased, it rejected the more balanced teachings of Christ. So women found it increasingly difficult to practice medicine or, indeed, any profession. Some women did of course manage to circumvent the railings of the Church; in Celtic Britain there were many revered and highly skilled women physicians. Sadly, however, no records exist of these women healers, and we have to study the myths of that culture to gain an insight into how women practiced medicine in those days.

## Queen Isolt of Ireland

Isolt practiced medicine and became famous throughout Ireland for her healing skills. At that time England was a subject nation to Ireland and had to send a tribute of young men each year to the Queen of Ireland as a tax or levy. One year a young nobleman called Tristram was chosen to be sent. He rebelled against this decision and, before being forced to leave for Ireland, fought a duel with Isolt's brother, Morhaut. In the fight Tristram was badly wounded, but Morhaut died. The tip of Morhaut's sword was poisoned, and Tristram's wound immediately began to fester and give off an awful stench. The Irish told him that he must seek out Isolt, and she would cure his terrible wound.

Tristram became an outcast because of his evil-smelling wound. In desperation he decided to travel to Ireland to find Isolt. He disguised himself as a harpist and sailed there. The Irish, a nation of bards and songsmiths, received him warmly, and his fame quickly spread throughout the whole of the country. Queen Isolt came to hear about this legendary harpist and summoned him to her court to teach her his harping skills. When he arrived at her court, she could not stand the stench of his wound and sent for her daughter, also named Isolt, to heal his wound:

> And all that day she lay him on a plaster, and anon the stench came out of the wound and the night next after the Queen took the wound with her own hand and washed it out with healing balms and bound it with marvellous plasters so that within short space she did away the swelling and the venom. In all the world leech was there none so knowing of all manner arts of healing, for she could know to help all manner diseases and wounds wherewith men may be visited. She was cunning in the virtues of all herbs that may be used unto any good, and wist all devices and means that pertain unto leechcraft. She knew thereto how to give succour against poisonous drink, and to heal poisonous wounds and perilous pains and all manner swellings, and to draw the smart out of all limbs, so that nowhere was to be found one more skilled nor of leechdoms a better master.[8]

Tristram recovered from his terrible wound by the healing ministrations of these two women.

## Morgan le Fay

Morgan le Fay is another legendary character. As high priestess of Avalon she presided over the Celtic mysteries associated with King Arthur and the knights of the round table. She is believed to have been one of the last priestesses of the old religion. In her book *The Mists of Avalon*, Marion Bradley describes how gradually, under the hand of Guinevere, Arthur's queen, Christianity took hold in Britain and many of the old ways were outlawed. Her book gives a moving account of the struggle between two world views and relates how Christian attitudes, beliefs, and values took over, not by reasoned argument but by repression and fear.[9]

Morgan le Fay was a priestess-healer similar to those in ancient Egypt and classical Greece. Her role was to concern herself with the welfare of her flock in physical, mental, and emotional domains. This meant a thorough knowledge of surgery and prayers to the goddesses of healing. Malory's *Morte d'Arthur* describes how she healed some of Arthur's knights and even Arthur himself.[10] Druidic bards carried by word of mouth the myth of Avalon and Morgan le Fay. In time, the story became corrupted by the Christians, and Morgan le Fay was cast in the role of a wicked, cunning witch who plotted Arthur's downfall, a far cry from that of a noble priestess.

Two written records that relate the healing methods of the time survive from the Dark Ages. *The Leech Book of Bald*, written around 300 C.E. but believed to have been derived from material of a much earlier date, and the *Lacnunga*, also dated around the tenth century and clearly pagan in origin.[11] Both books must have been written for physicians, for few people at that time could read; even many monks and nuns were illiterate. From the recipes and charms set out in these books it can be seen how far medicine had changed from the sophisticated practices of the Greeks and Egyptians. The following charm, a spell to heal a wound, is taken from the *Leech Book of Bald*:

> *I have wreathed round the wounds*
> *The best of healing wreaths*
> *That the baneful sores may*
> *Neither burn nor burst,*
> *Nor find their way further*
> *Nor turn foul and fallow*
> *Nor thump and throle on,*
> *Nor be wicked wounds,*

*Nor dig deeply down;*
*But he himself may hold*
*In a way to health*
*Let it ache thee no more*
*Than ear in Earth acheth.*

This charm "serves" for one with "water elf disease" in which a person would have livid nails and tearful eyes and would look downward. The herbs to use would be: yewberry, lupin, helenium, marshmallow, dockelder, wormwood, and strawberry leaves.[12]

The *Lacnunga* is altogether a more poetic work and describes the healing properties of the number nine. The following excerpt is in praise of the nine sacred herbs: mugwort, waybroad (plantain), stime (watercress), atterlothe, maythen (chamomile) wergulu (nettle), crab apple, chervil, and fennel.

*These nine attack*
*against nine venoms.*
*A worm came creeping*
*he tore assunder a man.*
*Then took Woden*
*Women Healers*

*Nine magic twigs,*
*then smote the serpent*
*that he in nine [bits] dispersed.*
*Now these nine herbs have power*
*against nine magic outcasts*
*against nine venoms*
*& against nine flying things*
*against the loathed things*
*that over land rove.*
*Against the red venoms*
*against the runlan [?] venom*
*against the white venom*
*against the blue venom*

*against the yellow venom*
*against the green venom*
*against the dusky venom*
*against the brown venom*
*against the purple venom*
*against worm blast*
*against water blast*
*against thorn blast*
*against thistle blast*
*against ice blast*
*against venom blast.*[13]

As the Christian church increased its hold, the pagan holistic no-
tions of medicine were discarded and the schism between matter and
spirit grew. The church taught that the body as flesh represented all
that was evil and corrupting, base and unspiritual. Medicine naturally
suffered as a result; its status and that of its practitioners reached
rockbottom. Since according to Christian doctrine women were wicked,
the combination of woman and healer was perceived to be diabolic.
Although there was no active persecution of women during these
times—nothing like the wholesale slaughter that was to follow—
nevertheless the status of women declined dramatically with the growth
of Christianity.

## St. Bridget

St. Bridget (453–525) was a woman healer in Ireland. It is not clear
whether or not she actually existed or was made over by the Christians
to be an example of a Christian saint. She is probably related to the
pagan Brigit whose festival was celebrated on the Celtic day of Imbolc
(1 February). The Irish called her Mary of the Gel, and she, together
with St. Patrick, were said to be the columns on which Ireland rested.
In pagan times the inexhaustible fires of Brigit were tended by twenty
virgins surrounded by a circular hedge of bushes into which no man
could enter. If a man did venture in, divine vengeance would occur. It
was a healing sanctuary; lepers were cured there, the lame left walking,
and the blind had their sight restored. The Bridget of the Christians

was said to have been the daughter of a druid priestess. She was converted to Christianity and practiced both midwifery and medicine. She worked in County Kildare, tending the impoverished and the sick.

## Eudoxia

In 420 the Empress Eudoxia, wife of Theodosius, founded a hospital in Jerusalem and also established two medical schools, one in Syria and the other in Edessa (Mesopotamia). She was a Nestorian Christian, a follower of St. Nestor, and practiced a gentle, loving Christianity. The established Pauline branch of the church wanted the Nestorians out of Edessa as they were perceived to be a threat to the patriarchal, woman-hating followers of St. Paul. Eudoxia moved the Edessa school to Persia where the queen (whose name is not recorded) welcomed her and accorded her and her followers every facility. Eudoxia sent to Greece for medical texts and the school established a great reputation. The empress Eudoxia personally funded the translation of many medical texts and opened clinics for the poor and needy.

## Radegonde

Radegonde was a princess of Burgundy. She was given as a prize of war to King Clothaire (497–561) who took her as his fifth wife. Outraged and desperate at her fate, she resisted the king in all ways open to her. She undertook to study medicine and opened a hospital for lepers in the palace precincts. She attracted the poor, the lame, and all the beggars of the area around her. She wanted to escape her marriage and become a nun (often the only way out for noble-born women), but the local bishop was afraid of the king and his legendary bad temper and refused her request. Clothaire was deeply insulted by the fact that his wife wanted to be rid of him and ordered the killing of Radegonde's brother as a punishment and warning to her. She fled Clothaire's palace and, in 542, hid in a convent in Poitiers, which had been founded by a friend of hers, Cesaria. Eventually the bishop, under constant pressure, gave way to Radegonde's demand to become a nun, and she settled in the Abbey of the Holy Cross, which housed both monks and nuns. This was an enclosed order, which meant that the nuns were forbidden to communicate with the outside world. Radegonde eventually became abbess, and under her guidance the abbey became a center for learning. It was supported financially by the rich women in the area and later by Clothaire who finally became reconciled to his wife's decision. Radegonde herself sold all her jewels to finance the building of a hospital. She trained over 200 nuns in the art of healing, and when she died in 587, hundreds flocked to her funeral. Miracle cures were said to have occurred at her tomb.

Religious orders took over much of the work of healing. Nunneries and monasteries housed dispensaries and medicinal herb gardens from which they took herbs to make their remedies. Any treatment would have an additional religious component, and relics or rosaries and the saying of prayers would be used in conjunction with the wearing of talismans and charms to keep away "devilish influences."

## Hilda of Whitby

Hilda of Whitby (614–680) was another nun and physician who carried on the ancient tradition of priestess-healers. She was born an Anglo-Saxon princess, being the niece of Edwin of Northumbria. Hilda converted to Christianity and was consecrated in what is now known as Hartlepool. She became abbess of the convent there in 648 and was the first nun to have been trained in Britain. In 657 she built her abbey at Whitby, where for thirty years she taught and practiced medicine, theology, grammar, music, and all the known arts. She trained five bishops and was a leading light of the new church. She was a skilled healer and personally took charge of the sick who came for treatment to the hospital she established in the convent grounds.

## Mildred

Mildred, another abbess living in the seventh century, was given lands by Egbert of Kent to found a convent. Within its grounds she opened a hospital for the local poor and is reputed to have cured hundreds of parishioners with her medical skills. She was revered and almost worshiped by those who came in contact with her. When she died, the dust from her tomb was used as a medical potion to cure a variety of illnesses.

In the eighth century when the Moors conquered Spain, they trained indigenous Spanish women in their healing arts, in particular midwifery and alchemy, both Arabic specialities. The Islamic social and religious belief that no male physician could attend a woman necessitated the training of these women.

The medical school in Baghdad was said to have had 6000 pupils of both sexes. There were also flourishing schools in Cordoba, Cairo, and Toledo. The great Arabic physician Rhazes (860–932), who had so much influence on European medicine, acknowledged he was jealous of the talents of women physicians and freely admitted he often learned new remedies from them. He said women had little medical knowledge but great insight and by using kindness and optimisim, often succeeded where men had failed. He noted they had great humility, much more than men.

# 3

# Trotula of Salerno

No woman physician has aroused such controversy as Trotula of Salerno. She has been called many different names, including the first woman professor of medicine and a crazy old midwife. Since the sixteenth century, historians and midwives have been debating, proving, and disproving her existence. They have both praised and dismissed her work.

## THE ATHENS OF THE TWO SICILIES

Salerno was and is a famous spa and health resort near Naples in southern Italy. Known as the Athens of the two Sicilies, the city was sacred to Phoebus, nurse to Minerva, and a meeting place for merchants, scholars, invalids, and crusaders, as well as brigands, pirates, Vikings, and other marauding bands. Originally settled by the Greeks, it was taken by the Norman conquerors and adopted as a home for Arabic students who flocked to its schools. They eagerly shared their medical, chemical, and alchemical knowledge with the Jews who quietly copied the manuscripts into many languages.

In the Middle Ages Salerno was famous for its climate, mineral springs, and physicians. It was known as the Hippocratic city. The sick, the poor, and the lame flocked to its doors in search of cures. The place became a famous healing center, and its hospitals had a worldwide reputation.

The medical school at Salerno was universally recognized as the "day star," the best of the European medical schools because of the thorough instruction given there. It revived the teaching of Hippocrates whose works were translated in many an attic in the old seaport, Salerno being an international market for medical and scientific manuscripts that arrived in the ships docking at the harbor. It was a cultural melting pot. A three-year course in philosophy and literature was required before a student could enroll in the medical school, and once enrolled, the student underwent a long and thorough training and took rigid examinations. The course in medicine lasted five years, after which time clinical practice with a physician was required.

Salerno tolerated women scholars and their practice. The medical school was the only one at that time that opened its doors to women, as well as to Jews and Moslems. The famous *Mulieres Salernitanae* (women of Salerno) were trained at the university. They were women physicians and were believed to have been professors in the theory and practice of medicine.

## THE TROTULA DEBATE

The most noted and successful practitioner among the women of Salerno was Trotula. It is said that she lived during the eleventh century, although her date of birth remains unknown. She was believed to have occupied the chair of medicine at the School of Salerno, as well as to have run an extensive clinical practice. She was the author of many medical works, and she and her husband both contributed to the encyclopedia of medicine, *Regimen Sanitatis Salernitanum,* one of the most popular medical works of the time.

No other woman physician has aroused such debate or such high feeling. Many male physicians are convinced she was a man, or else fictitious. Women who have researched her life, however, among whom are Kate Campbell Hurd-Mead, Elizabeth Mason-Hohl, and Margaret Alic, provide convincing evidence to support the claim that Trotula was a woman and author of the words ascribed to her.

Given that history, until very recently, has been recorded by white, male, middle-class Christian writers, it comes as no surprise that these historians considered the existence of a woman of such high standing to be very unlikely, if not downright unbelievable. Trotula was, after all, one of the foremost authorities on medicine for hundreds of years, whose extant works were published and republished many times and were bestsellers. Margaret Alic[1] suggests that she might have been the Trotula who joined her husband and two sons on the School of Salerno faculty after it was reorganized in the middle of the eleventh century and worked with her husband on the *Practica Brevis*, which the medical school produced.

## WORKS ASCRIBED TO TROTULA

The most famous of the written works ascribed to Trotula is *Passionibus Mulierum Curandorum (The Diseases of Women)*, which begins with the phrase *cum auctor*, by which it is often referred to in academic discourses. This work is also known as *Trotula Major*. Part of the problem in accepting that this text was written by an eleventh-century woman is the intimate and often explicit nature of its contents. The descriptions of female anatomy and sexuality have made male historians disbelieve that a woman could have written them. Nineteenth-century historians especially had trouble reconciling the rugged and frank discussions of sexual behavior in the light of their contemporary understanding of women. As John Benton says, "[medieval] men knew little about feminine physiology and some were intensely troubled by their ignorance."[2] He describes a story of a man who discovered his abdomen covered with blood after having sexual intercourse and became frightened because he did not know why this was so.[3] Male physicians did not make intimate examinations of female patients, neither were they present at childbirth, so they would not have had direct access to the information contained in Trotula's book. She wrote it to educate male medics about the workings of the female physical body. Margaret Alic observes:

> Trotula's straight-forward descriptions of the diseases of celibacy
> and sex seem to have offended the Victorian-minded historians
> of the early twentieth century. . . . But medieval readers had no
> difficulty with frank discussions of sexuality.[4]

Trotula's other book, *De Aegritudinum Curatione* or *De Ornatu Mulierium,* is more of a cosmetic recipe book. It was also known as *Trotula Minor.* This work includes treatments for scrofula, lice, and various lesions. At some point in time the two texts, *Major* and *Minor,* were combined, and what is usually referred to as "Trotula" is the combination of these two works. This is all that remains of her work.

Salvatore de Renzi, who wrote about medicine in Salerno in the nineteenth century, claimed that only a fragment of her work remained and that the majority of her clinical and medical writings had been lost. Pascal Parente, writing a century later, echoes this point of view: "Only fragmentary chapters remain today of Trotula's voluminous writings."[5] Herman Rudolf Spitzner [6] gives the names of nineteen manuscripts of Trotula, dated in the thirteenth century. These are to be found in the libraries of France, Germany, Belgium, Austria, Oxford, and Cambridge.[7]

Trotula is mentioned in Chaucer's *Canterbury Tales.* The husband of the wife of Bath describes the book her husband read when he had the "leyser and vacacion"; it was a volume containing Tertullum, Trotula, and Helowys.

A story survives of a wandering minstrel of the thirteenth century who tells his tale to an assembled crowd:

> good people, I am hardly one of you itinerant preachers, one of those raggle taggle herbalists ... who carry boxes and sachets and spread them out on a carpet. No, I am a disciple of the great lady named Trotula of Salerno, who performs such marvels of every kind. And know ye that she is the wisest woman in the four quarters of the world.[8]

A thirteenth-century scientific encyclopedia talks about: "physicians who know nothing, derive great authority and much solid information" from Trotula, partly "because she was a woman, and all women revealed their inner thoughts more readily to her than to any man and told her their natures."[9]

The gynecology in Trotula's work reflects some progress in contemporary practice, especially regarding the instructions for repairing a lacerated perineum and the need for support of the perineum in pregnancy. Likewise her professional, rather than emotive, outlook regarding sensitive matters such as abortion, show the handling of gynecology and obstetrics to be an integral part of a *magistra's* practice. John Benton takes up the argument:

> a striking feature of the three treatises which have traditionally been attributed to Trotula is that they were so frequently copied and so widely disseminated. The existence today of nearly one hundred manuscripts shows that they became the standard gynaecological texts of the late medieval medical profession.

And he continues "no one doubted that these treatises were written by a woman."[10]

Modern sceptics include Charles and Dorothy Singer, well-respected researchers in the history of medical and scientific writing in the early twentieth century. They attempted a literary reconstruction of the medical school at Salerno and proposed that Trotula's work was written by Trottus, a man, and that Trotula was simply a miscopying of his name. They claimed that Trotula was the name for his collected works, which was a common practice in Italian medical schools.

> The first woman professor has been deprived of more than her chair by the unchivalrous mythoclasts. . . . The good wife Trotula passed long ago into the fairy-tales as "dame Trot." Alas she too had no existence.[11]

But their attempts to belittle Trotula's contribution to women's medicine have been vigorously opposed by a great many women doctors. As Kate Campbell Hurd-Mead says:

> To any woman doctor of the twentieth century, therefore, there would seem to be no good reason for denying that a book having such decidedly feminine touches as TROTULA'S was written by a woman. It bears the gentle hand of the woman doctor on every page. It is full of common sense, practical, up-to-date for its time.[12]

# TROTULA'S MEDICAL WRITINGS

My source for Trotula's medical writings is *Passionibus Mulierum Curandorum,* translated by Elizabeth Mason-Hohl—the page numbers referred to in the quotes are from this book.[13] It is the first English translation of the Aldine version of 1547 and was included in a version of *Medici Antiqui Omnes,* a compilation of the thirteen greatest medical authorities of early times, from Stabus Gallus (63 B.C.E.) to Trotula.

Trotula's first consideration when encountering a sick person was his or her comfort. She believed in treating patients gently, giving them medicated baths and suitable diets. Fires were lit if the house was cold and damp. Patients' faces were sprinkled with sweet-smelling extracts. For example, Trotula recommends oil of roses for foul-smelling ulcers. In her treatment of the sick, simples (that is, herbs boiled in syrup) were given, which were colored differently for different diseases. She believed in long convalescences; above all, wherever possible, she gave a hopeful prognosis. Remedies were prescribed with faith and hope, for even in her times psychology was the handmaiden of medicine.

The book comprises sixty-three chapters, the first on regulating the menses and on the significance of heavy and light blood loss. The problems of conception, pregnancy, and childbirth are dealt with in detail, and there is a section on general diseases. The book ends with the preparation and formula for an elixir of life. The majority of remedies are herbs, spices, and natural oils. Sometimes Trotula prescribes remedies made from animals. The testicles of a wild boar or pig, for example, are powdered and mixed with wine and drunk at the end of a menstrual period to help a woman conceive (p. 19). This is clearly a hormonal treatment for sterility as the testicles contain the hormone testosterone, which can be used to regulate hormonal balance.

Trotula combines the scientific with the magical. Her prescription to prevent conception has a touch of the spell maker's practice:

> lay on the last afterbirth as many grains of cataputia or of barley as the years which she desires to remain sterile. If she wishes to remain barren forever let her lay on a handful (p. 19).

The majority of the remedies are simple, commonsense healing remedies, together with gentle caring nursing practice. In one section, Trotula describes how she went about her work and discovered what remedies were appropriate for which conditions. The following case comes from chapter 20, entitled "On incidents which befall women after childbirth." In this episode Trotula describes her work as an applied scientist as well as physician healer.

> Once a certain girl who was afflicted with flatulence of this sort suffered as if from rupture. When I saw her I became interested to the utmost degree and made her come into my own house that I might in secret learn the cause of the sickness.
>
> When I learned that the pain was not from rupture or swelling of the womb but from flatulence I had a bath made for her of cooked mallow and shredded wool. I put the patient into it and treated those parts frequently and sufficiently by softening them. I had her stay in the bath a long time and when she came out of it I made a poultice for her of the juice of bearded *tapsum*, wild rape and barley flour. I applied this hot to clear up the flatulence. Later I made her stand in the bath and so she became cured (pp. 29–30).

Trotula goes into a great deal of detail about ailments and recipes for the newborn. She discusses the factors which hinder conception. Certain women, she maintains, cannot conceive because they are either too fat or too thin. Some have wombs that cannot retain seed, or the semen of the man is too thin and slips out of the uterus. "It is evident therefore that conception is hindered as often by a defect of the man as of the woman" (p. 16).

This was radical thinking indeed in eleventh-century Italy. The "woman as vessel" was seen as responsible and culpable for any malfunctions associated with childbirth. The man caused the fetus to come into being, but the woman was its "curator." So to admit that the man might also be responsible for infertility was a daring and very challenging step.

Concerning male sterility Trotula notes:

> if conception be hindered because of a defect of the male it
> would be from a lack of force impelling the sperm, a defect of the
> organ, or a defect of heat.... If it happens through a defect of the
> sperm the sign is that when he copulates he emits either none or
> too little seed (p. 18).

In such an instance she recommends items that increase sperm, such
as orris root and domestic parsnip. She also provides a test to decide
whether it is the man or the woman who is infertile. Two jars should
be filled with bran and the urine of the man should be put in one of
them and that of the woman in the other. They should be left for eight
or nine days. If a person is infertile, the bran in his or her jar will be
foul and have many worms. If, however, there are no worms in the
bran, that person is fertile (p. 18).

Trotula's understanding of the role and function of male sperm was
by no means widespread, and it is significant that it echoes modern
thinking relating to the viscosity of seminal fluid and sperm count in
male fertility treatments. Trotula also describes the changes in vaginal
mucus that occur at ovulation. The mucus becomes more fluid and
allows the sperm to swim up the vaginal canal more easily. She describes
how this mucus can be too slippery and therefore unable to "hold" the
seed. Likewise, if the womb is too hot, it cannot provide a favorable
environment for the fetus to develop, and miscarriage will occur.

The physiology of the body is described from the viewpoint of the
four elements, or the system of the four humors, which was described
by Galen, although it was in use for centuries before his accounts were
written.[14] Trotula writes:

> He [God] made the nature of the male hot and dry and that of the
> female cold and wet so that the excess of each other's embrace
> might be restrained by the mutual opposition of contrary quali-
> ties. . . . Since then women are by nature weaker than men it is
> reasonable that sicknesses more often abound in them especially

around the organs involved in the work of nature. Since these organs happen to be in a retired location, women on account of modesty and the fragility and delicacy of the state of these parts dare not reveal the difficulties of their sicknesses to a male doctor. Wherefore I, pitying their misfortunes and at the instigation of a certain matron, began to study carefully the sicknesses which most frequently trouble the female sex (pp. 1–2).

Trotula outlines her reasons for undertaking the study and practice of medicine, which are reminiscent of Agnodice in first-century Rome. She was "called" to the art and science of medicine, having seen women suffering from gynecological and obstetrical diseases because they felt too ashamed and embarrassed to talk to a male doctor. She had a much more positive viewpoint and describes the monthly blood loss as a purge, cleansing the body. She calls the menses "flowers," because "just as trees do not produce fruit without flowers so women without menses are deprived of the function of conception" (p. 2).

Trotula quotes Galen and Hippocrates in the text, showing her familiarity with their works. This indicates she was a woman of some erudition, not simply an empirical practitioner. For example, she observes that Galen says that women who have narrow vulvas and light wombs ought not to have husbands lest they die if they conceive. Her understanding of physiology is further illustrated as she discusses the process of development of the embryo:

In the first month occurs a small clot of blood. In the second occurs the formation of blood out of the body and of the body; in the third the nails and hair are produced. In the fourth motion and therefore women are nauseated. In the fifth the foetus receives the likeness of father or mother. In the sixth, the binding together of the sinews. In the seventh the bones and sinews are strengthened; in the eight nature helps and the child puts on flesh. In the ninth it proceeds from darkness to light (pp. 19–20).

Trotula also gives sensible advice for a woman when she becomes pregnant:

care must be taken that nothing be named in her presence which cannot be had because if she shall ask for it and it not be given to her she has occasion for miscarrying (p. 21).

Modern findings showing that emotional traumas can cause miscarriage, especially in the first three months of pregnancy, back up this advice. When the hour of birth arrives, she has further advice. She recommends that the woman's abdomen be massaged with oil of violet and the diet consist of light, digestible foods. In her care of women giving birth, Trotula's profound psychological insight is revealed: "Let the woman be led with slow pace through the house. Do not let those who are present look in her face because women are wont to be bashful in childbearing and after the birth" (p. 23).

She quotes Hippocrates who recommended that if a woman has strange cravings, if she asks for chalk or coals, let beans be cooked in sugar and given to her (p . 21).

In her management of labor and advice for midwives, Trotula shows that she is more than a midwife and has the obstetrician's skill in turning the child:

> If the child does not come forth in the order in which it should, that is, if the legs and arms should come out first, let the midwife with her small and gentle hand moistened with a decoction of flaxseed and chickpeas, put the child back in its place in the proper position. If the child be dead take rue, mugwort, absinth and black pepper and give this pulverized in wine or in water in which lupins have been cooked. Or let savory be mashed and bound over the abdomen and the foetus, whether dead or alive, will come forth (p. 23).

She continues:

> Those who are in difficult labour must be aided in the following manner. Let a bath be prepared and the woman put in it; after she has come out let a fumigation be made of wheat and similar aromatics for comforting and relaxing. . . . Let sneezing be provoked with mouth and nostrils shut. . . . Also let those things

be done which have been mentioned before for bringing forth menstruation. If difficulty in childbirth should result from tightness of the mouth of the womb, the cure of this is more difficult than anything else. . . . Let the woman take care the last three months in her diet that she so use light and digestible foods that through them the limbs might be opened (pp. 24–25).

Such foods as egg yolks, meat, and the juice of chickens and small birds, partridges and pheasants should be provided.

In her care of the newborn, Trotula recommends that the eyes be covered and that special care should be taken that the baby is not in bright light. She suggests that the infant's ears be pressed into shape frequently. The navel cord should be tied measured three fingers from the abdomen.

Let there be in front of him varied pictures, cloths of various colours, and pearls. In his presence one should employ songs and gentle voices and no one should sing with a harsh voice. Nor should there be noisy persons about. When the time for the baby to talk has come, the nurse should frequently anoint his tongue with honey and butter. . . . Frequent and gentle words should be spoken in front of him. . . . When the time shall come when he begins to eat, cylindrical fingers the size and shape of an acorn should be given to the infant. He can hold them in his hand and play with them and sucking from them he will swallow some of it (p. 26).

Discussing postpartum, Trotula says "the womb like a wild beast of the forest wanders to this side and that because of sudden evacuation, thus producing violent pain" (p. 28).

For rupture of the uterus she recommends dried root of black briony and cinnamon and suggests these should be made into a powder and injected into the vulva (p. 28).

For expulsion of the afterbirth, Trotula says to: "take a root of rock parsley and leaves of leek. We draw out the juices, mix with a little oil and give it to the patient to drink. Then we lay vinegar on the vulva, and the afterbirth will come out" (p. 29).

Trotula's work was not simply gynecology; she also discussed in detail clinical diagnoses of various ailments. Urine was used as a diagnostic tool; there were twenty-nine observations to be made, based on color, smell, and composition. The pulse gave indications as to the state of the circulation and the heart. The color of the face, the condition of the eyes, and the feel of the skin were all used to determine the cause of the sickness. Death could be forecast by five signs, and there were three types of disease: inherited, contagious, and self-generated. Diagnoses were precise. Trotula was, for example, able to differentiate between malaria and typhoid and to calculate the height of the fever and the date of recovery. Dysentery, she claims, sometimes comes from yellow bile and sometimes from phlegm (p. 41). The treatment for the latter is thyme flowers; for dysentery caused by bile she recommends red roses in rainwater. Silk or cotton should be dipped into the mixture and applied to the anus.

Trotula taught her students to be observant:

> When you reach the patient, ask where his pain is, then feel his pulse. Touch his skin to see if he has a fever, ask if he has a chill, and when the pain began, and if it was worse at night. Watch his facial expression, test the softness of his abdomen and ask if he passes urine frequently, look carefully at the urine, examine his body for sensitive spots and if you find nothing ask what other doctors he has consulted and what was their diagnosis, ask if he had ever a similar attack and when. Then having found the cause of his trouble it will be easy to determine his treatment.[15]

Hurd-Mead claims that Trotula was the first author to write about pediatrics as a separate branch of medicine. Her use of opiates to dull the pain of childbirth was strictly against the teaching of the church, which maintained that women should suffer the pangs of childbirth without any relief.

Trotula provides a comprehensive and far-reaching example of medieval medical practice as seen from the viewpoint of a woman practitioner. That her interest should be to alleviate the suffering of women shows clearly that she speaks from the viewpoint of a woman who understands what it is to be a woman.

# 4

# Hildegard of Bingen

SAINT, MYSTIC, HEALER, VISIONARY, FIGHTER, Hildegard of Bingen stands as one of the great figures in the history of women in medicine. She wrote profusely on a wide variety of subjects, more than any other woman of her time. And this is a period of history when few women could write even a letter. She was a friend and correspondent of popes, emperors, and queens and was renowned and respected for her healing work and her original theories of medicine. She was also a well-respected and talented artist, poet, musician, and composer.

## HILDEGARD'S LIFE

Hildegard was born in Bermersheim in the beautiful German province of Rheinhessen in 1098. She was the tenth and last child of a noble and well-connected family. She claimed that from the age of three she was subject to visions, which did not come to her in her sleep but in her waking hours; yet they were not heard with the ears or seen with the eyes.

When she was eight years old, she was sent to the monastery of Disibodenberg to spend her life in the enclosed order of anchoresses. She was put in the care of Jutta of Sponheim. An anchoress was required to stay in her cells until her death, with no hope of leaving. As it was a life of such strict enclosure, it was seen to be a sure way of obtaining everlasting bliss, hidden from the world for good, for the glory of God. The ritual performed by the monks to enclose an anchoress was similar in form to that of the burial rites.

The anchorage at Disibodenberg was under Benedictine rule as the adjoining monastery was of that religious order. The anchorites learned the psalms by rote; psalters were the universal primers of the Middle Ages and were often owned and read by laywomen. Hildegard was taught to read by Jutta the abbess, who took charge of the young girl's education and whom she much loved. Music formed an early part of this education. Hildegard was raised on a frugal diet and was simply clothed. She would eat one meal a day in winter and two a day in summer, comprised of vegetables or fruit and bread. No meat was eaten from four-footed animals except by the sick and very weak. The main diet consisted of beans, eggs, fish, and cheese.

Hildegard was tutored by a monk, Volmar, one of the *magisters* (masters) of the adjoining monastery. She later collaborated with him in the writing of her books and the recording of her visions. The first book they worked on, *Scivias (Know the Ways of God, or The Book of Faith)*, was a rendition of her visions. She was very strict about how Volmar transcribed the visions; he was allowed to change only the grammar in the text, not to alter its substance. Volmar was provost in charge of the spiritual welfare of the nuns, and he and Hildegard became close friends. It was to him she turned when her visions started to come with increasing frequency.

Gradually, the anchorite order grew. As more and more women came to the anchorage, it changed from being a closed order to an ordinary Benedictine nunnery. At fifteen Hildegard was invested as a Benedictine nun. Her education continued with Volmar, who un-doubtedly taught her medicine as the Benedictines were renowned for their medical skill.

When Jutta died, Hildegard became the administrative head of the abbey and was elected *magistra* (head) in 1136 at the age of thirty-nine.

As the majority of Hildegard's works were written in Latin, they were available only to a religious elite since few people outside the church were able to read this language. Hildegard would have been considered one of the intellectuals of her time. The prescribed course of education at that time included the study of grammar, not only Latin syntax but the study of classical literature, followed by rhetoric and dialectic and then the quadrivium, which consisted of music, arithmetic, geometry, and astronomy. This was followed by the study of theology or canon law or medicine. Women in Germany were not permitted to study in universities, so the only possibility of higher education came within religious orders.

One way in which the voice of women could be heard was as a prophet. A lack of education was not seen as an obstacle. As E. Petroff illustrates:

> Visions led women to the acquisition of power in the world . . . [they] were a socially sanctioned activity that freed a woman from conventional female roles. . . . They . . . gave her the strength to grow internally and to change the world, to build convents, found hospitals, preach, attack injustice and greed, even within the church.[1]

Hildegard was ordered in one vision, in 1141, to disclose the content of her visions. And from that time on she began to record and organize them with the help of Volmar. In 1147 she wrote to St. Bernard of Clairvaux (a leading figure of Cistercian reform) for advice about her visions. He spoke to Pope Eugenius II who sent two delegates to visit her and to take a copy of her as yet unpublished *Scivias*. Eugenius was so impressed by the work he personally read it to the delegates at the Synod of Trier in 1147. The council was also impressed, especially as Bernard expressed his belief in their authenticity. Eugenius wrote to Hildegard giving her apostolic license to continue writing, and from that time onward her fame began to spread, although Lynn Thorndike claims that: "her medical skill contributed more to her popular reputation for saintliness than all her writings."[2]

As news spread of this new prophet of God, an increasing number of postulants came to the nunnery, and their number grew to such an extent that it became clear they had to move. Hildegard had a vision that spoke clearly of the need to find another home for her and her followers.

In 1150 Hildegard moved to the new abbey at Rupertsberg with twenty nuns. She tried to gain financial independence from the monks at Disibodenberg, but the early years were times of hardship and it was not until 1158 that she obtained a charter regulating the distribution of assets between the two religious houses.

Life at Rupertsberg followed the counsel of Hildegard's visions, and the conduct of the nuns was considered bizarre, if not outrageous, for the times. They developed their own style of dress and worship and wore tiaras or crowns, believing that women should celebrate the celestial divinity. Hildegard saw visions of women clothed in gold and wearing crowns studded with gems interwoven with roses and lilies. This, she claimed, enabled the wearer to hear the harmonious music of heaven. The convent admitted only women of noble birth. Hildegard saw the human hierarchies as ordained by God; people were ranked like angels to be equally loved but not to be confused. Hildegard was a musician and a composer, and she saw music as a way of sharing in the life of heaven itself, the music of the heavenly spheres, the soul symphonic. Life at the abbey had an intensely mystical flavor. They even had their own special language (over 900 words of which survive) which described things of everyday use: clothes worn by the nuns, herbs, natural and heavenly things. Hildegard lived out her visions.

## HILDEGARD'S WRITTEN WORKS

Hildegard's works were hard to read as her writing style was complex. Her two medical works are full of German expressions, which are absent from the prophetic works.[3] Hildegard, however, made no claim for divine inspiration for her medical work but saw the two texts, *Causae et Curae* and *Subtilitates*, as extensions of her experience and practice of medicine.

*Causae et Curae* is a medical compendium, divided into five books. The first begins with the creation of the universe and the fall of Lucifer. The second deals with celestial phenomena: Adam, Eve, and the flood. There follows a discussion of natural phenomena. In Book Three the medical texts begin. She spoke of those who walk the path of truth and discussed how the four elements held the world together and how they form the structure of the human body.[4]

She took an essentially pragmatic view of medicine, recommending a balanced diet, rest, and the alleviation of stress, together with a wholesome moral life. For example, she maintained that if our deeds are just, the elements will hold their course; if not, our conflicts will affect our hormonal balance and thus our physical health, which is Hildegard's explanation of how the psyche affects our bodies, or psychosomatic medicine. In *Causae et Curae* she says passions such as wrath and petulance affect the body.[5] She continues:

> Just as the four elements hold the world together they also form
> the structure for the human body. . . . Fire, air, water and earth
> are in human kind, and humans consist of them. From fire they
> have their breath, from water they have their blood and from
> earth their bodies.[6]

She describes the four humoral types thus:

> **De sanguinea** [Sanguine types] Some women are inclined to
> plumpness and have soft and delectable flesh and slender veins
> and well-constituted blood free of impurities. . . . And these have
> a clear and light colouring, and in love's embraces are themselves
> lovable; they are subtle in arts, and show self-restraint in their
> disposition. At menstruation they suffer only a moderate loss of
> blood, and their womb is well developed for childbearing, so
> they are fertile and can take in the man's seed. Yet they do not
> bear many children, and if they are without husbands, so that
> they remain childless, they easily have physical pains; but if they
> have husbands, they are well.

> **De flecmatica** [Phlegmatics] There are other women whose
> flesh does not develop as much, because they have thick veins
> and healthy, whitish blood (though it does contain a little impu-
> rity, which is the source of its light colour). They have several
> features, and are darkish in colouring. They are vigorous and
> practical and have a somewhat mannish disposition. At men-
> struation their menstrual blood flows neither too little nor too

abundantly. And because they have thick veins they are very fertile and conceive easily, for their womb and all their inner organs, too, are well developed. They attract men and make men pursue them, and so men love them well. If they want to stay away from men, they can do so without being affected by it badly, though they are slightly affected. However, if they do avoid making love with men they will become difficult and unpleasant in their behaviour. But if they go with men and do not wish to avoid men's love-making, they will be unbridled and over-lascivious, according to men's report. And because they are to some extent mannish on account of the vital force [*viriditas*, literally greenness] within them, a little down sometimes grows on their chin.

**De colerica** [Choleric types] There are other women who have slender flesh but big bones, moderately sized veins and dense red blood. They are pallid in colouring, prudent and benevolent, and men show them reverence and are afraid of them. They suffer much loss of blood in menstruation; their womb is well developed and they are fertile. And men like their conduct, yet flee from them and avoid them to some extent, for they can interest men but not make men desire them. If they do get married, they are chaste, they remain loyal wives and live healthily with their husbands; and if they are unmarried, they tend to be ailing.

**De melancolica** [Melancholic types] But there are other women who have gaunt flesh and thick veins and moderately sized bones; their blood is more lead-coloured than sanguine and their colouring is as it were blended with grey and black. They are changeable and free-roaming in their thoughts, and wearisomely wasted away in affliction; they also have little power of resistance, so that at times they are worn out by melancholy. They suffer much loss of blood in menstruation . . . and thus they are also healthier, stronger and happier without husbands than with them—especially because, if they lie with their husbands, they will tend to feel weak afterwards. But men turn away from them and shun them, because they do not speak to men affectionately, and love them only a little. If for some hour they experience sexual joy, it quickly passes in them. Yet some such women, if they unite with robust and sanguine husbands, can at times, when they reach a fair age, such as fifty, bear at least one child. . . . If their menopause comes before the just age, they will sometimes suffer gout or swelling of the legs, or will incur an insanity which their melancholy arouses, or else back-ache or a kidney-ailment. (Translated by Peter Dronke, pp. 180–1.)[7]

Although Hildegard suffered because of her culture's low opinion of women, she saw wisdom as the *creatrix* and the *anima mundi* or *sapientia* who created the world by living in it. Thus her spirituality was of the world; holistic, inclusive of all that was natural and beautiful, seeing the holy spirit or the divine in everything. She did not see the flesh as sinful nor as less of a work of God than the mind, for example. This was against the teachings of the church, which preached the sinfulness of things material, earthly, and worldly and the need to castigate or flagellate the flesh into submission.

Like Trotula, Hildegard the physician was deeply sympathetic to women and to the ailments they suffered from and, like her, she called the menses "flowers" or the fruit of the womb. Woman's menstrual flow was Eve's river of blood, the ground of her fertility, so the pain of menstruation should be an occasion for mercy and not for judgement. She said:

> I do not disdain this time of suffering in woman, for I gave it to Eve when she conceived sin in the taste of fruit. So a woman during her period should be treated with the great medicine of mercy.[8]

The divine voice also gave menstruating women the right to attend church, but denied this right to men wounded in battle. Eve's wound was God-given and therefore sacred, but wounds of battle were man-made and came from sin.

Hildegard's psychosexual writings on women have led many readers to doubt her authorship. Like Trotula, later scholars could not imagine that a woman might write with such openness about sexuality. But, any working physician, which Hildegard clearly was, would come in contact with a variety of complaints and issues. And being a woman physician, women patients would tell her things no male physician would ever discover:

> When a woman is making love with a man, a sense of heat in her brain, which brings with it sensual delight, communicates the taste of that delight during the act and summons forth the emission of the man's seed. And when the seed has fallen into its place, that vehement heat descending from her brain draws the seed to itself and holds it, and soon the woman's sexual organs contract, and all the parts that are ready to open up during the time of menstruation now close, in the same way as a strong man can hold something enclosed in his fist.[9]

Nevertheless there is an ambivalence in Hildegard's writing about sexuality. Christian tradition was overwhelmingly hostile to sexuality in general and women's sexuality in particular. Yet at the same time both Christian and Arabic texts of that time were able to treat sexuality calmly without ethical considerations. But there remained woman's mystical nature, which longed to part with the physical world and to transcend nature, and the pragmatic sensualist, who loved beauty and all of God's creations. Unlike contemporary theological dogma, Hildegard believed in the purity of women and claimed that most women would remain celibate if they had the choice. She argued that women were colder than men, that they represented the body while men represented the soul. But she saw the earthly complexion as male, due to Adam's formation from the earth and airy temperaments. Women's temperament was more sensitive to the physical environment, retaining the ethereal nature of Eve. This, she claimed, affected woman's passion; she was more able to restrain desire, because of either fear or modesty.

Pleasure in woman is like the sunlight, which mildly, gently and continuously suffuses the earth with its warmth to make it fruitful, for, if it burned more keenly in its constant blaze, it would injure the fruit instead of helping it grow.[10]

Hildegard believed that although most women would rather remain virgins, virginity required a special vocation. She saw women's bodies as being like lyres. In *Causae et Curae* she writes about intercourse and conception using Galenic ideas. Fire by its dryness kindles the will; air moves consideration beyond measure; water causes the power to surge; and earth makes consent. All the humors arouse a tempest, which draws from the blood a poisonous foam, semen, which unites with women's blood. She believed it remained poisonous until it was united or neutralized by the womb. "It remains a poisonous foam until fire or heat warms it, air or breath dries it, water or fluid dampens it with pure moisture, and earth or skin confines it."[11]

She said if a man's seed was strong a male child would be born, and if weak, a female. The child would be virtuous if the parents cherished each other at the time of conception, but if love was lacking on one side or the other, the offspring would be weak. If it was lacking on both sides, the child would be bitter. Although *Scivias* contains a polemic against astrology,[12] a lunar horoscope was appended to *Causae et Curae*, which has been both refuted and accepted.[13] Hildegard emphasizes the influence of the moon and, as Thorndike puts it, "in which respect she resembles many an astrologer."[14] She says that some days of the moon are good, others bad, some useful and others useless, some strong and others weak and that human blood and the brain are augmented when the moon is full and diminish as it wanes. She suggested that sometimes epilepsy occurs when there is an eclipse of the moon[15] and counsels that men should respect the phases of the moon when planning a family.

One who is conceived on the first day after the new moon, when it receives its splendour from the sun, if a boy he will be proud and hard, and love no man except one who fears and honours him . . . he will be healthy in body and have no great sicknesses, though he will not grow very old. If a girl is born, she will always covet being honoured, and will be loved more by outsiders than by her household.[16]

Conception was seen as fortunate in the waxing moon as both the blood and semen, a product of blood, increases with the increase of the moon. In Book Five of *Causae et Curae,* Hildegard lists astrological prognostications and predictions for each day of the month.

In the section on gynecology she lists herbal concoctions such as salves, potions, plasters, and baths. She compiled this list from her own observation and her knowledge of over 200 plants, as well as animals, gems, and what nowadays would be called sympathetic magic. Her science had a Greek background, which used Galenic and Aristotelian theories altered to bring them in line with the scriptures. She never used Arabic medical terms and was probably not acquainted with the works of Avicenna. Trotula's work, however, would have been available to Hildegard as it was widely distributed at that time.

Hildegard avoided the topics of contraception and abortion as both were vehemently opposed by the church, but she does include recipes for "retention of the menses," a polite term for abortifacient. One such recipe involved constructing a type of sauna, using fresh river water, heated tiles, and a bouquet of "warm" herbs such as tansy, chrysanthemum, feverfew, or mullein. The woman had to sit in the bath so as to cover her navel to "soften her flesh and womb and open up the constricted veins."[17]

Cold retains the periods, so when there is pain, the woman should bind the thighs with linen dipped in water or ivy warmed in water. A gentle massage of the limbs and trunk should follow.

Like Trotula, Hildegard sees the problem of infertility as one affecting both sexes. In the male, the semen may have been too fluid, the womb too cold, or, in the final analysis, a judgment of God. If it is a problem of the woman, Hildegard recommends eating the womb of a sexually mature but virgin calf before (or during?) sexual intercourse. The succulent juices will moisten the womb, and the pure animal's fertility will be transferred to the woman.

Hildegard saw labor pains as part of the curse of Eve. She believed that Satan set out to ambush women during labor and she advised the wearing of amulets to protect the woman and child. Jasper and fern are two she recommends. She suggests a moist poultice of fennel and hazelwort and that the woman carry a red carnelian (a gem) and stroke her thighs with it saying: "As you, jewel, shone by the command of God in the first angel, so you, infant, come forth as a shining man abiding in God." The patient then had to hold the jewel over her vagina and recite the following charm: "Be opened, passages and portal, in the name of that epiphany by which Christ appeared as God and man and opened the gates of hell; that you, infant, may go out at that portal without your own or your mother's death."[18]

At that time, gemstones were widely employed in healing. They were seen to be fiery in nature and were associated with the fire of the spirit and the fire in which Satan burns. They were used for honor, blessing, and healing. They reminded the devil of his lost beauty, and because of their innate virtue, they could only be used for honorable ends.

Hildegard believed that humanity was essentially good and that our sins show how we have distorted the good. She was inspired by the spirit of goodness, of balance and moderation, and the need to live in harmony with the elements to keep an internal harmony so that health is maintained. She called it *viriditas* (greenness) and said it was like the vital force, mother earth, and the rational soul, which were behind all life. Dronke refers to it as "the earthly expression of the celestial sunlight; greenness . . . is the . . . overcoming of the dualism between earthly and heavenly."[19]

*Physica* consists of nine books divided in sections. The first book is a collection of 200 short monographs on plants, minerals, trees, jewels, birds, animals, and metals. Plants are described as hot or cold. For example: "Dornella (tormentil) is cold, and that coldness is good and healthy and useful against fevers that arise from bad food. Take tormentil therefore, and cook it in wine with a little honey added . . . and drink it fasting at night and you will be cured of the fever."[20]

Trees are the subject of the third book which relates their relative heat and coldness to the size and quantity of fruit produced. Those producing large, abundant fruit are hotter than those with small, sparse fruit. Many tree remedies should be collected before the fruit appears. Apples may be eaten raw except by the sick. Like plants, trees are characterized by heat and coldness. Both the box and the fir trees are exceptionally hot and she recommends them to keep away evil spirits. And from Book Three chapter 28 comes a remedy for babies:

> If any baby lying in its cradle is suffused and vexed with blood between the skin and flesh so that it is greatly troubled, take new and recent leaves from the aspen and put them on a simple linen cloth and wrap the baby in the leaves and cloth and put him down to sleep, wrapping him up so he will sweat and extract the virtue from the leaves, and he will get well.[21]

Hildegard also described the properties and virtues of fish at great length, probably because she lived near a large river. They formed an important part of the diet, for example, from chapter 22: "a freshly caught herring is not good for man to eat since it might make him swell up . . . but when it has been soaked in much salt and will hurt him less." She goes on to describe the medicinal uses of animals, for example, a lion's ear is a cure for deafness but the leopard has no medicinal uses. Hildegard also discusses minerals such as gold, silver, lead, and tin. Fevers, for example, were treated with copper boiled in wine.

Hildegard held the view, common at that time, that the purpose of the natural world was to illustrate the spiritual world and the life to come, that invisible and eternal truths are manifested in visible and temporal objects. They represent the divine and also the diabolical. In *Causae et Curae,* chapter 25, she discusses a powder to be used "against poison and magic words." It also confers health and courage and prosperity on him who carried it with him.

> First one takes a root of geranium with its leaves, two mallow plants, and seven shoots of the plantagenet. . . . These must be plucked at midday in the middle of April. Then they are to be laid on moist earth and sprinkled with water to keep them green for a while. Next they are dried in the setting sun and in the

rising sun until the third hour, when they should once more be laid on moist earth and sprinkled with water until noon. Then they are to be removed and placed facing south in the full sunshine until the ninth hour, when they should be wrapped in cloth, with a stick on top to hold them in place, until a trifle before midnight. Then the night begins to incline towards day and all the evils of darkness and night begin to flee. A little before midnight, therefore, they should be transferred to a high window or placed above a door or in some garden where the cool air may have access to them. As soon as midnight is passed, they are to be removed once more, pulverized with the middle finger, and put in a new pill box with a little bisemum to keep them from decaying but not a sufficient quantity to overcome the scent of the herbs. A little of this powder may be applied daily to the eyes, ears, nose and mouth, or it may be bound on the body as an antiaphrodisiac, or it may be held over wine without touching it but so that its odour can reach the wine, which should be drunk with a bit of saffron as a preventative of indigestion, poison, magic, and so forth.[22]

Thus Hildegard's magic was as superstitious as the devilish arts she condemns. But her beliefs were in accord with the times in which she lived. Christianity was fiercely opposed to anything which smacked of the devil, and yet employed the same means, using different forms than those of which heretics and witches were accused.

Hildegard the mystic is well illustrated in the introduction to *Causae et Curae* where she writes,[23] "O man look to man. For man has the heavens and earth and other created things within him. He is one, and all things are hidden within him." A profound spiritual truth that all is contained within ourselves should we trouble to look for it, God himself (or the goddess) lives inside us, all we need is patience and faith to look for our divinity. Hildegard discusses the divinatory nature of dreams and says that God sent sleep to Adam before he sinned. His soul saw many things in true prophecy and sometimes the human soul can do the same thing, though it is too often clouded by diabolic illusions.[24] But when the body is in a temperate condition and the marrow warmed there is no disturbance of vices and the sleeper sees the true dreams. Such were the visions of Hildegard. Her divine insight gave her life a depth and richness and breadth of vision which encompassed the physical sciences and healing, as well as the spiritual, metaphysical realm.

> I am a remedy [medicine] for all the conditions you have caused. I heal where you destroy. I declare all these things, such as wars, as unjustified, self-defeating, and an everlasting contention. I am a mountain. . . . I am full of fragrance like myrrh and incense.[25]

# 5

# $\mathcal{W}$omen Physicians in the Late Middle Ages

FROM THE TWELFTH CENTURY ONWARD, a series of both natural and man-made disasters changed the fabric of European society.

The most deadly was the bubonic plague, which was brought into central Europe by the Goths and Huns. Those who died in their millions were city dwellers; peasants in the country survived the epidemics better because of their relatively more sanitary living conditions. The plague had a devastating effect on the cultural and intellectual life of those living in Europe. The previous flowering of art, music, and other cultural pursuits came to a dramatic halt, and medicine suffered likewise. Superstitions, the saying of prayers, and the use of incantations, religious relics, and the wearing of amulets replaced sensible hygienic measures and became just as prevalent as in the Dark Ages. The standard of living was reduced to subsistence level as famine fueled the fires of the plague and the malnourished population succumbed easily to this foreign disease.

In the middle of the thirteenth century the Black Death arrived from Sicily and spread rapidly through Italy, France, and the Low Countries. It has been estimated that from one third to one half the population of Europe died from the Black Death. It is hard to imagine the terror and despair of the population as it spread like a brush fire through towns, cities, and villages. Church records show that in only three days 1500 people died in Avignon, while the Franciscan order claimed that over 124,000 lives were lost in this first outbreak.[1] By 1350 the population of Europe had been reduced to half of what it had been only ten years previously.

For some reason, women seemed to survive the plague better; in some areas their recovery rate was about seven times that of men.[2] This caused widespread fear and resentment, and men began to suspect that women were using diabolic means to survive the illness and to cause the death of their menfolk. The Black Death returned again and again. In 1478 it killed a third of the population, which had already been decimated by previous outbreaks of the plague. Also in 1478, a form of syphilis, which had been dormant for over seven hundred years, resurfaced.

Europe was also embroiled in numerous wars, which further reduced the population and ruptured the fabric of society. For instance the Hundred Years' War between Britain and France started in 1346, while the Wars of the Roses in England lasted from 1455 to 1485.

The Crusades, which began in 1099, also totally disrupted the lives of people in Europe. It is estimated that 800,000 people died in the First Crusade, with similar numbers of casualties in the Second and Third Crusades. While these holy wars were fought, life in the home countries deteriorated as there were no men to grow crops or to carry on traditional crafts.

On the one hand, women had more freedom than they had had for many centuries, especially while the men were away fighting the wars. They were left to run estates and businesses and go about their lives as they pleased. But the only occupations open to women were obstetrics, surgery, pharmacy, and teaching. All these professions had the low status associated with women's work. As Kate Campbell Hurd-Mead said: "These occupations were somewhat scornfully left to women provided they were not too conspicuously successful in them."[3]

But as the death toll rose, life became increasingly difficult, and women were not well equipped to survive the ravages of war and famine. The burden of nursing and healing fell to the women. Uneducated and for the most part unskilled, they carried out their medical work as best they could, while at the same time they were severely punished if they were found practicing medicine.

By the thirteenth century all university places were closed to women and Jews, with the exception of those in Italy. When the men returned from the wars, women were once again treated like chattel. They were seen as a threat to the status quo by the returning soldiers who expected life to be as it had been before.

## Anna Comnena

King Alexis of Constantinople built a vast hospital in Constantinople in 1081, which was reputed to have more than 10,000 beds. The king passed the administration of the hospital over to his daughter, Anna Comnena, who was physician-in-charge. She wrote a book about the treatment of gout and also compiled a treatise on the history of her father's reign called the *Alexiad,* which mentions her medical under-standing. It is clear she was trained by some of the finest physicians of her time, as the following quotation illustrates:

> It seems to me if a body is sickly, the sickness is often aggravated by external causes, but that occasionally, too, the causes of our illnesses spring up of themselves, although we are apt to blame the inequalities of the climate, indiscretion of diet, or perhaps too, the humours as the cause of our fevers.[4]

Comnena mentions many kinds of illnesses, using her contemporary Galenic understanding of medicine. She made a connection between envy and gangrene, for example, seeing the powerful emotion as having a physical effect.

## Bertha

Bertha, Anna's sister-in-law, built a larger hospital, the Pantocrator, in 1126 to house wounded pilgrims from the west. A woman doctor ran each of its five sections, and the work was divided between midwives, male and female nurses, and surgeons. At one time the hospital was run by an English woman, Edina Rittle of Essex.

## Eleanor of Aquitaine

In spite of absolution having been granted to women and children who stayed at home, many thousands left with their menfolk to fight the infidel and remove him from Jerusalem. Few ever returned. In the second crusade in 1145, the women in this ragtag army were led by Queen Eleanor of Aquitaine (1122–1204), at that time wife to Louis VII of France. She founded hospitals all along the route taken by the crusade. A legend in her own lifetime, Eleanor was later to marry Henry II of England. Mother of ten children, her sphere of influence at one time extended from the Orkney islands in Scotland to the Pyrenees. She was a fine scholar and was one of the most learned women of her age. Eleanor gave birth to a dynasty of women healers.

## Isobel

Eleanor's daughter, Isobel, was noted for her medical skills. She founded the nursing order the "Poor Clares," who devoted their lives to the sick and dying. They transformed their nunneries into hospitals for the sick and dying, grew their own medicinal plants to make medicines, and had their own pharmacies.

## Hedwig

Isobel's granddaughter, Hedwig Queen of Silesia, Poland, and Slavic Croatia (1174–1243), was convent educated. After having six children, she decided to live a celibate life and devote herself to charity. She built hospitals, tended the sick in clinics, and had feeding programs for the hungry and destitute. She and her family built over 18,000 asylums for lepers in her realm. She was canonised in 1267.

## Blanche of Castile

Blanche, the granddaughter of Eleanor of Aquitaine, built a beautiful gothic hospital at Royaumont, about twenty-five miles from Paris, which still stands. Her son, Louis IX (Saint Louis) "took the cross," and she ruled his kingdom as regent. In his name she founded a school for surgeons in Paris and built many other hospitals and monasteries.

## Isobel

Blanche's daughter, Isobel Queen of Sicily, built a gothic hospital at Tonnerre near Dijon in 1293, which, like that of her mother, is still standing.

## St. Elizabeth

St. Elizabeth of Hungary was a niece of Hedwig. Born in 1207, she was betrothed at the age of seven. Her education was overseen by her aunt, and she studied medicine at the Wartburg near Eisenach. At fifteen her marriage was consummated, and she had four children before the age of twenty. Her husband went to fight in the Crusades and never returned. Elizabeth was treated badly by her husband's family and left in impoverished conditions with her four children. Elizabeth set about doing healing work in her castle in Kreuznach, training the local women in nursing skills, binding wounds, soothing fevers, and easing pain. She died at the early age of twenty-four and was canonised for her selfless efforts.

## Hersende

Louis IX appointed Hersende of the Abbey Fontevrault to be *maitresse physicienne* for the Seventh Crusade. Hersende saw to his queen's confinement in Egypt as well as overseeing the medical and surgical work with the sick and wounded soldiers and camp followers.

Jewish women in Europe dominated the medical profession from the twelfth to the fifteenth centuries, despite the increasing discrimination they suffered and a ruling by the church that they were forbidden to treat Christians. It was recognized that they were superior physicians; often multilingual, they had access to the medical writings of the great classical medical writers, including Trotula, Cleopatra, and Hildegard. Jewish women physicians worked with Arabic women throughout the vast Moorish Kingdom. Because of the strict rules of Islam, Muslim men refused to have their women attended by male physicians and were also unwilling to educate their women, so they trained Jewish women to attend them. Slave girls to the harems also often had superior medical knowledge and many were house physicians. The following story translated from *The Thousand and One Nights* illustrates the level of scholarship to be found in these women.[5] Tawaddud was the slave of Abu al-Husn of Baghdad. He had terrible debts, and to help him out she suggested that he should sell her. She said they should gather together all the great minds of that city to put her learning to the test, and whoever could better her could buy her for an exorbitant sum. She knew so much medicine that no one could better her: she had studied Galen, astrology, the humoral theory, and the seven liberal arts, as well as Aristotle and the Talmud. None of the learned physicians gathered there could outwit her. One famous doctor remarked: "this damsel is more learned than I in medicine. . . . I cannot cope with her."[6]

Tawaddud even triumphed over the rhetorician Ibrahim, outwitting him. She was finally bought for a great price but as a reward set free. She chose, however, to return to her old master.

Jewish itinerant doctors traveled across Europe and the Middle East, escaping the persecutions and pogroms. They often found work translating medical texts from Arabic, Latin, Hebrew, and Greek. Many settled in the busy seaport of Salerno which was a center for the exchange of medical literature. Jews were considered to be the best eye doctors and surgeons. Jewish women specialized in obstetrics and gynecology and used techniques taught by the women of Salerno. They were familiar with many techniques unknown to other physicians such as how to use a vaginal speculum and how to perform cesarean sections.

## Marie of France

When Eleanor of Aquitaine returned home from the crusades, she paid many troubadours to entertain the people of France. One, Marie of France, lived in the French court and wrote songs to accompany her lyre. She told of the wonderful medical women of Salerno, their famous remedies and their poisons, and sang of Salernian medicines that could bring the dead to life and, according to Kate Campbell

Hurd-Mead, showed: "considerable medical knowledge in her descriptions of the diseases and wounds for which these remedies were used by the women doctors of her times."[7]

Among the Parsifal tales in Germany are stories of women travelling to Salerno for medical advice and tuition. In the German epic *Gudrun* (written about 1250), we are told of "wild women," that is, self-taught medical women from Russia who taught magic and the healing arts to Queen Wate, along with love potions, emmenagogues (medicines to abort), poisons, and antidotes.

In the *Sturlunga* saga of Iceland the lives of the women of the Sturlunga family are recorded (1116–1264). They patched up wounds, engaged in building hospitals, and tended the sick. In one story, a woman, Svanhvit, finds her husband wounded in battle; she sews up his wounds and sends him back healed to fight again.

## Jaqueline Félicie de Almania

Jaqueline Félicie de Almania, also known as Jacoba Felice, was Jewish and born in Paris around 1280. She received medical training and began practicing in Paris in the first half of the thirteenth century. She was treated badly by jealous colleagues and found herself indicted under threat of excommunication on 11 August 1322. The charge was that she was illegally practicing medicine and she was brought before the bishops of Paris and the Proctor and Dean of the Medical Faculty of Paris University.

The charges laid against her were that she visited many sick persons suffering from serious illnesses in Paris and the suburbs. She examined their urine, felt their pulses, and examined their bodies. After examining their urine she was reputed to have said "I will cure you by God's will, if you will have faith in me." She would then make a compact for the cure and would receive a fee. Following her compact, she would cure the patient of internal illnesses and external wounds. She would visit the sick assiduously and continue to examine the urine "in the manner of physicians," feel the pulse and touch the body and limbs. Then she would give the patients syrups and potions, laxatives and digestives, aromatics and other remedies, which they would drink in her presence according to her prescription. She practiced in Paris and the suburbs, although she had not studied at the schools of Paris and was therefore not licensed. She had been admonished by decree of venerable official men of Paris under pain of execution and fined sixty Parisian pounds. In spite of these charges, however, she continued to visit the sick and administer medicines as before.

John of Padua, who had been surgeon to the King of France, Philip IV, was a witness for the prosecution. He argued that the laws prohibiting and excommunicating illicit empirics had been in operation for more than sixty years, that Jaqueline knew only too well she was acting contrary to the law, and that she had persisted in practicing medicine, although she was ignorant of the art and not educated or competent in those things she presumed to treat. He argued that through her ignorance she might easily kill someone, that such a death would be a mortal sin, and that thus she should be excommunicated.

The defending counsel had equally emphatic arguments. It was shown that Jaqueline had treated and cured many sick people. She had comforted her patients when others had failed to do so and had visited and cared for them assiduously until they were cured. This was corroborated by the many witnesses brought forward by the defense counsel. The court asked each witness how he or she had heard of Jaqueline, whether she had presented herself as a qualified practitioner, whether she had tried to extort money, and whether they knew that she was not qualified. All the replies were similar. They had learned of her through a friend; she had proceeded as most physicians had by taking a case history and doing a diagnosis. She had refused to take any money until the patient had been cured, so they had not enquired about her qualifications. One of the witnesses, John of St. Omar, said she had cured him of an illness and had visited him several times. She had done more for him than any other physician. She had made him a remedy of a clear-colored liquid. His wife, Matilda, attested the cure and also added that Jacqueline had applied poultices to her chest. Another witness, John Faber, said she had cured him by giving him two potions, one of them green and one clear.

A female patient, Yvo Tueleu, related how she had been ill with a fever and several physicians had visited her, none of whom had been able to cure her. At her request, Jaqueline had come to her bedside and had given her a purgelike remedy, which had cured her of the fever. Another patient, Dominus Odo de Cornessiaco, a friar at the Hotel Dieu, said he had been treated by several notable physicians but that none had been able to cure him. He then consulted Jaqueline who had given him steam baths, massages with oil, and poultices with chamomile, meliot, and other plants. He claimed she had worked without stopping until he was cured. The testimonies carried on in this vein.

The counsel for the defense also argued that there were many people practicing in Paris without a license. He went on to attack the legality of the stature of the university. The law was invoked by the medical faculty, but it had no legal validity as it had not been approved by medical practioners not associated with the university. It was meant only as a warning to unlicensed practitioners who were ignorant of medicine.

In summing up, the defense counsel asserted the decree of the faculty of medicine could not be binding as it went against the public good.[8] The defense quoted a speech made by Jaqueline, which incorporates the arguments of most women healers:

> It is better and more seemly that a wise woman learned in the art should visit the sick woman and inquire into the secrets of her nature and her hidden parts, than a man should do so, for whom it is not lawful to see and to seek out the aforesaid parts, not to feel with his hands, the breasts, belly and feet of women. And a woman before now would allow herself to die rather than reveal the secrets of her infirmities to a man.[9]

The university, however, regarded these arguments as inconsequential and found Jaqueline guilty of willful disobedience. She was excommunicated from practicing medicine and from exercising the functions of a physician.

It is a terrible indictment of male-dominated medicine that the charges brought against Jaqueline were not those of malpractice or extortion. Neither was there any suggestion that she was a bad physician. Jaqueline's only crime was her sex; as a woman she could not graduate in medicine and thus she was guilty. Part of her sentence reads as follows: "Her plea that she cured many sick persons whom the aforesaid masters could not cure, ought not to stand and is frivolous, since it is certain that a man approved in the aforesaid art could cure the sick better than any woman."[10]

## Christine de Pisan

Christine de Pisan was another famous French woman who put her thoughts into rebellious poetry. Born the daughter of the French court astrologer in 1364, she expressed her discontent in literary works. She was a feminist who talked about the harshness and ingratitude of men who debased and devalued women, even though these women spent their lives caring for their men.

> *Heavens what assemblies*
> *Where the honors of women are stolen!*
> *And what profit comes thus from defaming [women]*
> *To those very persons who ought to arm themselves*
> *To protect them and defend their honor.*
> *For every man ought to have tender regard*
> *Toward woman, who is a mother to him*
> *And is not changeable or bitter to him,*
> *Always gentle, sweet, and amiable,*
> *To his needs sympathetic and helpful;*
> *Who performs many serviccs for him,*
> *And from whom many deeds are designed*
> *To nurse the body of a man tenderly;*
> *To her master, in life and death,*
> *Woman is helpful and comforting,*
> *Piteous, sweet and serviceable*
> *And he is lacking in understanding and is rude*
> *Who slanders her, and full of ingratitude.*[11]

Christine de Pisan advocated the education of women so that they might be able to manage their own affairs, treat the sick, and perform operations when necessary. In despair one day she prayed to God that he turn her into a man, and he replied by showing her a vision of a city of women in which they all lived happily and were ruled by reason, righteousness, and justice. She had her own medical and philosophical theory; it posited the existence of seven elements of the body, seven healing remedies, and seven forms of treatment: purges, evacuants, tonics, heating and cooling remedies, and bleeding and thinning medicines. Although not a physician, Christine de Pisan understood the plight of women physicians and was herself well versed in the medicines of the day.

# 6

# The Struggle to Practice: Women Healers Under Threat

## WOMEN'S POWER

Matilda Gage, who began the feminist analysis of the witch craze in the nineteenth century, claims that the "witch was in reality the profoundest thinker, the most advanced scientist of those ages. The persecution which for ages waged against witches was in reality an attack upon science at the hands of the church."[1]

For a thousand years, the witch was the only physician of the people. The emperors, kings, popes, and richer barons had the doctors of Salerno, then the Moors and the Jews, but the general population consulted none but the sages or wise women.[2]

> A vast amount of evidence exists to show that the word "witch" formerly signified a woman of superior knowledge. Many of the persons called witches [were able] . . . to heal by a touch. . . . Many were doubtless psychic sensitives of high powers . . . able to perceive the hidden principles of all vegetable or mineral substances. . . . Besides the natural psychics who formed a large proportion of the victims of this period, other women with a

natural spirit of investigation made scientific discoveries . . . the one fact of a woman possessing knowledge served to bring her under the suspicion and accusation of the church.[3]

Such women would have been intuitives, healers, masseurs, herbalists. They would have worked with nature, gently encouraging the vital spirit, rather than attacking disease with powerful, deadly remedies. They would have prescribed painkillers and anesthetics to mitigate the suffering of women during childbirth and menstruation. This was in direct opposition to the teachings of the church, which taught that the pain women suffered during childbirth was Eve's curse and not to be interfered with. Those who sought to avoid this curse were believed to be working with the devil. As Matilda Gage states, much of the persecution was aimed at woman's

strong natural bias toward the study of medicine, together with deepest sympathy for suffering humanity . . . such women losing their lives as witches simply because of their superior medical and surgical knowledge.[4]

Throughout the centuries it has been universally accepted that women are healers. It has been understood that they have contact with a source of healing power above and beyond human understanding, which has been described as sorcery or the magic of women. These healing powers have been seen to be in some way connected with a woman's ability to create life and bleed in rhythm with the moon. There are numerous superstitions relating to menstruation, which transcend class, race, and culture.[5] Menstrual taboos show the fear and awe this blood loss creates in men and explains many of the blood rites that men have developed to imitate the menstrual blood loss of their womenfolk. Menstruating women are feared, pregnant women are worshiped, virgins are symbols of fertility and purity, and crones, that is, postmenopausal women, represent the dark chaos that is woman.

Shamans are trained to take on the illnesses of their patients and, by so doing, heal them. Before they can use these skills, however, they need to have experience of "other worlds," or different realities. They need to maintain a link with the supernatural spiritual forces to make a contract with the sick person and heal her or him. Women were seen to have more of a connection with these worlds, although the teachings of the church strenuously countered such beliefs. To the church, women were the embodiment of matter. They were perceived to be earthly, while men were believed to be closer to God and the holders and dispensers of spiritual truths. For most people, however, the reverse was true. Women were seen to have access to these supernatural realms. It was women who could hex and heal, using unseen forces. The church tried hard to quantify and regulate the natural world and order the spiritual world. Women were seen to be inherently more anarchic, fluid, and open and more willing to challenge and confront. To men with a rigid worldview, such freedom was both terrifying and dangerous. Women allowed for the possibility of chaos, upending the orderly world of medieval men. As such, women were seen to be a corrupting influence. They had the power to turn men's thoughts away from God and lead them to the devil.

## THE DOCTRINE OF ORIGINAL SIN

Men in medieval times, backed by the Christian church, set about debasing and belittling the power of women and taught of their inherent wickedness, their potential for causing harm. To steal women's power, the church created a mythology of their sinfulness and evil intent.

The temptation of Eve by the serpent and her subsequent fall formed the basis of the misogynist teachings of the church. However, the story of the Garden of Eden predates Christianity by thousands of years. In the original story, the queen of heaven, the ideal woman or spiritual mother, encounters the tree of wisdom and a serpent, which is an ancient symbol of female wisdom and the female mysteries. The serpent calls on her to deepen her knowledge and to take this wisdom into her body, to absorb it corporally. Christianity turned the symbolism of the myth on its head and made the serpent represent wickedness; it changes from a symbol of wisdom to one of the devil. In the Christian myth the serpent seduces Eve and encourages her to defy

God and eat from his tree of knowledge. This wisdom is for God alone, and she dares to usurp his authority, his rule. By so doing she corrupts man, dragging him down from heaven to her earthly level and all that is flesh. For this, the one God punishes her and curses her, so that she shall bring forth children in pain and sorrow and be subservient to her partner, man.

Woman is thus both the culprit and the corrupter, the tyrant and the victim. Paradoxically, woman is at the same time weak and helpless in the face of her temptation and yet an all-powerful malignant force, strong enough to counter all that is good, which is personified by man. It is she who seduces man from his lofty heights and drags him down to earth, to all that is base and defiled.

## THE WITCH CRAZE

Believers in the doctrine of original sin had few scruples about taming this she-devil. The church's teachings gave men license to act out whatever unspeakable brutalities came to mind. It gave carte blanche to torturers, sadists, rapists, and pedophiles.

> Her womb from her body. Separation. Her clitoris from her vulva. Cleaving. Desire from her body. *We were told that bodies rising to heaven lose their vulvas, their ovaries, wombs, that her body in resurrection becomes a male body . . . we were told that the blood of a woman after childbirth conveys uncleanliness . . . that if a woman have an issue and that issue in her flesh be blood, she shall be impure for seven days.* The impure from the pure. The defiled from the holy. *And whoever touches her, we heard, was also impure. Spirit from matter.*[6]

Beautiful as she was, her beauty was a mask to cover her terrible ugliness. The Book of Revelation describes woman as

> The great whore that sitteth upon many waters with whom the Kings of the earth have committed fornication, and the inhabitants of the earth have been made drunk with the wine of her

> fornication. . . . I saw the woman drunken with the blood of the
> saints and with the blood of the martyrs . . . and shall make her
> desolate and naked and shall eat her flesh; and burn her with fire.
> And in her found the blood of prophets, and of saints and of all,
> that were slain upon the earth.[7]

The church fed fear into the minds of men who then forced women through a reign of terror to heed church doctrine. It could not take away the life-bearing function of women, neither could it reduce their physical allure, but it could, through men, reduce women's activities and sphere of influence and stop them from working. Together with the legal profession and the physicians, the church sought to exclude women from medicine to curtail their freedom of movement in society and their access to the power and prestige a craft or profession would give. Male physicians were greedy for women's skills and the money to be earned from them. They sought to exclude women from the mainstream of life.

Death by torture was the church's method for repressing of women's intellectual knowledge, for it was held to be dangerous and evil in her hands. As the Bible states: "I do not permit a woman to be a teacher, nor must a woman domineer over a man; she should be quiet." (1 Timothy 2: 11–12.)

Women had a strong tradition in all aspects of medicine and at all levels, from the wise women in rural communities to professors in European universities. Their existence was common, if not widespread. Women were seen by men to be threatening and very powerful, and the fact that they had skills that were vital to the survival of the community would have naturally increased men's fear and suspicion.

> For, clearly, the intent was to break down and destroy strong
> women, to dis-member and kill the Goddess, the divine spark of
> be-ing in women. The intent was to purify society of the exist-
> ence and potential existence of such women.[8]

Within any community, anywhere in the world, the witch-healer is both respected and feared. Jeanne Achtenberg gives a chilling example of the fate of one woman healer. Alison Peirson of Byrehill had established a reputation as a gifted healer: "The Archbishop of St Andrews was suffering from an illness which the orthodox physicians could not heal. He sent for Alison and she healed him. After he was better, the Archbishop declared she was a witch, refused to pay her for her work and she was arrested and executed for witchcraft."[9]

## MIDWIVES UNDER ATTACK

Women throughout the ages have always had a monopoly in midwifery, and this became one of the many focuses of conflict between churchmen and women healers. It was said that: "No one does more harm to the Catholic faith than midwives."[10] And in 1554 Bishop Bonner declared that: "A mydwyfe shall not use or exercise any withcrafte, charms, etc."[11] If the charms were of the Christian variety, however, they were permitted. Women were told to bind a long charm in Latin on their thighs, beginning with the words: "In the name of the Father and the Son and the Holy Spirit," followed by an invocation to the saints and the secret names of God. This charm was said to protect women in labor.

In 1559 it was asked "whether you know anye that do use charmes, sorcery . . . or imaginatoris invented by the Devyl, specially in the tyme of women's travyle."[12] And in 1591 a Scottish noblewoman, Eufame Maclayne, was burned alive for asking a witch-midwife for drugs to ease her labor pains.

Babies delivered by midwives had to be brought to the church to be examined by the local priest for signs of bewitchment. The Archbishop of York advised that: "All curates must openly in the church teach and instruct the mydweifes of the very words and forme of baptisme."[13] There exists a record of a license given by the Archbishop of Canterbury in 1567 where a midwife was obliged to take a long oath and, among many promises, was to use the proper words at baptism and to use pure water to make the blessing, not rosewater or damask water.[14]

The church and the medical profession worked hand in hand to control midwives, and in certain districts of England the examination of midwives took place before both doctor and bishop. It was feared the women might sell the soul of the newborn infant to the devil before the church could claim it for its own by baptism. Midwifery was a lucrative business and some midwives became very wealthy as a result of their practices. Many doctors wanted to limit their activity so that they might cash in on the rich rewards.

All women involved in midwifery became targets. Their skills in diagnosis, healing, pharmacy, and divination were well known. Paracelsus, one of the great scientists of the Renaissance, said that he had learned much of his learning from women physicians. In 1527, perhaps frightened that he too might become a target for the wrath of the inquisitors, he burned his entire text on pharmaceuticals, declaring that "he had learnt from the Sorceress all he knew."[15]

## MALE PHYSICIANS UNDER THREAT

In everyday life male physicians were held in low esteem and were often seen as charlatans who charged large fees for common medicines. Bacon declared that: "Empirics and old women [were] more happy many times in their cures than learned physicians."[16] And another writer went even further to declare that: "Doctors of physic . . . were the greatest cheats . . . in the world. If there were never a doctor of physic in the world, people would live longer and live better in health."[17]

Male physicians, desirous of a more elevated position, ruthlessly denounced all opposition. The diagnosis of witchcraft was in the hands of both doctors and the clergy. The *Malleus Malificarum* states "for it cannot be cured by any natural remedy; or in the opinion of the physicians the illness is due to witchcraft."[18] With the Inquisition the doctor had tremendous power; he had the power of life and death. Once an illness was diagnosed as the result of bewitchment, the supposed witch was as good as dead. The clerics took over, enacting their sadomasochistic fantasies by raping and torturing the accused woman and her children.

If a disease existed, and male-dominated medicine could not cure it, then it was not a disease but rather witchcraft. If a woman should cure the illness, she was doing so with the aid of a diabolic agency and was therefore a witch. If the doctor gave medicine that aggravated the illness (by using a poison or wrong diagnosis, for example), he was not at fault; the patient was bewitched. The penalty for women presuming to heal, contrary to the teachings of the church and the knowledge of the medical profession, was torture and death.

So gradually women retreated. They backed away from practicing medicine in public, unless they were especially courageous or had the protection of a powerful man. Women scientists, scholars, healers, and physicians were forced to study alone and to hand down their knowledge orally, in secret and in fear.

Women's knowledge was not often written down and so was not available to men. This created a great deal of resentment and jealousy: "the combination of spiritual and medical knowledge made good witches the epitome of 'evil' to the Christian persecutors."[19] The church having forbidden its offices and all external methods of knowledge to woman, was profoundly stirred with indignation at her having through her own wisdom (and tenacity) penetrated into some of the most deeply subtle secrets of nature.[20]

## THEORIES ABOUT THE WITCH CRAZE

J. B. Russell[21] suggests that the causes of the witch craze are to be found in the church's campaign to put down heresy. He claims that witches, usually female, were part of a common heretical movement in the Middle Ages, that represented the mass of people who felt "deprived, not of wealth, but of the dignity and worth they deserved as human beings."[22] He maintains that women were actively engaged in the peasant revolts against the tyranny of the church, that the history of witchcraft had more to do with heresy than sorcery.

Gillian Tindall[23] believes that the witch cult was a relic of the ancient fertility cults that flourished in pre-Christian Britain and claims that such cults were far more attractive to women because of their matrifocal bias than the spiritual intellectualism of Catholicism. She concludes, however, that medieval women were essentially simpleminded and turned to the more eccentric fringe religions to counter the woman-hating dogma of the church. Quite apart from this misreading of pagan religion, Tindall attempts to make women culpable—albeit misguided, stupid, and deceived—by implying that these simpleminded women were responsible for their fate. She also decides that witches were always ugly—old and superfluous:

> I suggest that this sexual antagonism is one reason that persecution for witchcraft fell more . . . upon old women. The old woman is at last vulnerable. With her shaky, withered body and toothless gums she represents a cruel travesty of female allure . . . the resentful male may at last attack with impunity.[24]

Tindall, however, fails to take into account the rape, torture, and murder of women and girls, and it is suggested that a sexual and sadomasochistic force was at work in these tortures and ritualistic murders. As Mary Daly points out, rape was not considered to be torture. Neither were public stripping or other practices designed to humiliate and denigrate the accused.[25] And Walker maintains that: "It can hardly be doubted that a major driving force of all witch hunts was sadistic sexual perversion."[26]

Girls could be prosecuted at the age of nine-and-a-half. Women were tortured with pincers, pliers and red hot irons in the genitals and breasts. Imprisoned women were "visited" in their cells by zealous male Catholics—that is, they were raped. And this was known to be happening at the time. Peter Cantor, known as "Peter the Precentor," Rector of the Cathedral School at Paris, accused the Inquisition of falsely arresting "certain honest matrons, refusing to consent to the lasciviousness of priests."[27]

The inquisitors did not want people to know that women had been raped in prison, which was the usual practice of torturers and their assistants during the preliminary stripping, because the public had a curious double standard: the most outrageous torture was permitted but not sexual abuse. Inquisitor Foulques in Toulouse, for instance, was charged with arresting women for the sole purpose of raping them. Russell, in a précis of J. Glenn Gray's *The Warriors*, concludes that:

A man, like a brute, may rage in mindless destruction, but far more terrifying than brutalized soldiers are the sensualists of warfare, those who contemplate and luxuriate in their cruelty. Such men obtain sexual satisfaction, aesthetic pleasure, and delight in their destruction, rape, and killing.[28]

Gray, however, with great mental dexterity, claims that "the witch, like the sensual warrior, takes pleasure in corrupting all that a peaceful and just society holds dear."[29] This classic display of male doublethink is depressingly familiar.

The sexual theme is further corroborated by the understanding of what a spell or evil eye was and how it was believed to work. Charles Hoyt maintains that:

What is not generally recognized, however, is the sexual nature of this superstition. The charm ... is generally a phallus. ... "The Evil Eye" may be a sublimated expression of a very primitive anxiety indeed: the blind basic male fear of extinction in the vagina.[30]

Some writers go further in apportioning blame. The Reverend Zilboorg, for example, attempts to psychoanalyze the witch craze and comes up with some bizarre theories. He plants the blame squarely on women themselves and claims they were all quite mad: "the world, particularly the official world, was in a state of constant panic and those who thought they had good reason to be afraid, hopelessly confused human illness with sedition."[31] Zilboorg goes on to prove his theory with the case of Francoise Fontain who was accused of witchcraft in August 1291 in Louvier Normandy.[32] She had been working as a servant in Paris where she had been seduced (raped) by someone not known to her. Subsequently, she developed convulsions and auditory hallucinations. She believed she was possessed by the devil. She could not overcome her belief and was brought before the court where she had an attack of convulsions. She was ordered to have her head and the hair from her armpits shaved. This treatment "cured" her sufficiently so that the court did not have to proceed with the more drastic remedy of removing her pubic hair. Zilboorg, himself a psychiatrist, concludes that "It would be idle . . . to prove the obvious fact that she was a mentally sick girl."[33] Such a cure leaves a large question mark over the "sanity" of those who believed that a young girl might recover from the trauma of rape by having her body hair removed.

Christine Larner[34] claims that the witch craze was not a pagan cult of simpleminded old women, neither was it psychopathology, but simply a desire for revenge. She notes that "In situations of domestic stress and tension in which men resort to violence, women use witchcraft."[35] Cohn maintains that there existed the need within society for a scapegoat for the unacknowledged hostility to Christianity, and that the church "cynically and consciously" legitimized "an exterminatory policy which had already been decided upon."[36] There is undoubtedly a lot of truth in both these latter theories.

The Reverend Summers firmly believed that witches were an evil force and that the inquisitors were saving "society" (for society read men) from their wickedness. A witch, he maintained, was

> an evil liver; a social pest and parasite; the devotee of a loathly and obscene creed . . . a member of a powerful and loathsome obscene creed . . . a member of a powerful secret organisation inimical to Church and State.[37]

It is hardly surprising that men might suspect women wanted to change the way they lived. Women had no rights at all; they could not earn money or possess property, even the clothes they wore. Their children were not legally theirs.

I believe that the Inquisition was a carefully and cynically planned and executed assault on women who dared to move out of the narrow limits set down for them, especially in the field of medicine, where women were able to express their humanitarian tendencies. Men were afraid of the power and influence that women possessed and also of their possible rebellion against the patriarchal status quo. If women remained submissive, passive, and uneducated, they were left alone, but those few who managed to educate themselves and who set themselves up as authorities in their given subjects, and particularly those within the medical profession, had to be destroyed. Their intuitive and scientific knowledge meant they posited a real threat to inadequate and greedy male physicians.

## THE "NEW SCIENCE"

The "New Science" came in with the Renaissance and, together with its attitudes, beliefs, and values, transformed the worldview and the social fabric of European society. It did untold harm to the social and professional status of women.

Rene Descartes is credited with being the father of the new scientific thought and with saying "I think, therefore I am." As a philosophical statement it presents a chilling worldview. He does not say "I feel, therefore I am." Feelings are left out of his philosophy. Thought—cold, rational, logical, and analytical reason—replaces the softer, more inclusive intuition or sensing.

Descartes posited that the mind and body are separate entities, that the body is simply a machine without an organizing principle, and that the body can be understood if it is broken down into its component parts. He believed that mathematics is the key to understanding the workings of the universe. Each object, each phenomenon, can be analyzed and broken down into its component parts and explained using mathematical concepts.

The separation of mind and body and the leveling of all experience to that of the logical had serious implications for medicine. From the time of the Renaissance medicine changed from being an art to being a science. The numinous, unknowable mystery of life was discarded in favor of a cold, linear "life as a machine" philosophy, whereby organs and tissues of the body were dissected and viewed as entities in themselves. This lead to the position that medicine is in today. Molecular biology and nuclear medicine are the two modern specialties with the most funding and prestige. These two branches of medicine deal with the abstract, cold, and clinical side of medicine.

The "New Science" was studied at the new universities that came into being throughout Europe. They were, however, with the exception of those in Italy, all closed to women. Women, therefore, had no access to the new learning, unless they were wealthy enough to afford their own private tutors. So it rapidly became the sole preserve of men. And men used it to control and restrict women's activities.

The new scientists, far from distancing themselves from religion, embraced Christianity and incorporated the male god-father into their scientific imaginings of the role of woman in the heavenly scheme of things.

## THE RENAISSANCE VIEW OF WOMAN

While the Bible was a valuable source of woman-hating dogma, the ancient Greeks, whose work had become much more widely available with the invention of the printing press, also propounded a profoundly misogynist doctrine.

Both Pythagoras and Aristotle had put forward the notion that women were inferior to men. Pythagoras gave men and women the following attributes:

| MALE | FEMALE |
| --- | --- |
| limited | unlimited |
| odd | even |
| one | plurality |
| right | left |
| square | oblong |
| at rest | moving |
| straight | curving |
| light | darkness |
| good | evil[38] |

Aristotle maintained the purpose of nature was to create perfection and that men embodied perfection. Man's function was to implant semen in the female to produce more males. If conditions were not ideal, that is, the climate was adverse or the heat of the womb was incorrect, then an imperfect being, a female, would be born. Women were cold and this coldness limited their mental faculties because there was not enough heat in a woman's body to drive matter in her head, although paradoxically the brain was cold. Whereas a man was courageous, a woman was fearful; he was honest, while she was deceitful. A man had moral strength, while she had moral weakness. This naturally enough led him into temptation, so the man needed to subordinate the woman's wishes lest she should lead him into evil.

Aristotle suggested that a woman should subject her will to that of her husband, look after his property, keep strangers out of his house, be modest in her personal habits and dress, be tolerant of his moods and behavior, and, as if this were not enough, to keep her cold, wet brain busy, she was expected to pray for him in his absence. A woman did have some saving virtues: she was said to instruct man in the cult of love. Only virgins, however, could inspire men; sexually mature women were far more dangerous. Love was perfected by reciprocity, but the origin of love is beauty, of which woman has more than man. Other virtues were those that maintained her firmly in a subordinate position: long-suffering, humility, patience, compassion, and public charity. A Renaissance woman would have needed all these virtues to avoid the Inquisition's clutches and remain more or less sane.

*Gynaecea*, edited by three men and published in 1566, was a collection of ancient, medieval and contemporary writings on the theme of woman. It was an immediate bestseller. In the ancient texts, the Pythagorean view held sway. Aristotle said a male animal is one that generates in another, while a female generates in herself. She is passive, cold, moist, and desires completion through intercourse with the male.[39] Galen agreed with this, except that he maintained that female semen existed and had a role to play in the generation of children.[40] Kasper Hoffmann (1574–1648) maintained that the heat of a man's body gave him the attributes of courage, liberality, honesty, and moral strength. Hysteria, from the Greek *hysta* meaning womb, was an illness of women, causing lovesickness, melancholy, listlessness, and irrational behavior.[41] The vices of ambition, avarice, and lechery are associated with women.

A legal tenet of the times was that all women were understood to be either married or about to be married. Thus marriage:

is an immovable obstacle to any improvement in the theoretical or real status of women in law, in theology, in moral and political philosophy. Its influence is even apparent in medicine whence comes its "natural" justification.[42]

and:

Although apparently not bound by the authority of the divine institution of matrimony, doctors none the less produce a "natural" justification for women's relegation to the home and exclusion from public office, and provide . . . an important foundation on which arguments in ethics and politics and law are based.[43]

Or as the Bible states without any uncertainty: "It is better to marry than to burn" (1 Corr. 7:9).

# 7

# *W*omen Healers from the Sixteenth to the Eighteenth Century

FROM THE SIXTEENTH CENTURY ONWARD the status of women physicians declined rapidly. Herbalists were allowed to practice only if they could afford to buy the license from their local bishop. There was much quackery and a widespread distrust of doctors of every type. Registered practitioners were mainly concerned with bloodletting, whereas unlicensed women healers continued in their age-old traditions of preventive medicine, herbal remedies, and dietary therapy. As one man wrote to his wife:

> give the child no phisick but such as midwives and old women,
> with the doctors approbation doe prescribe; for assure yourselfe
> they by experience know better than any phisition how to treat
> such infants.[1]

Dr. Turbeville, a noted occultist in the West Country, was sent to cure the princess of Denmark who had a dangerous inflammation of the eyes. On his return he reported that:

> he expected to learn something of these Court doctors ... but he
> found them only spies upon his practice, and wholly ignorant as

> to the lady's case . . . he knew several midwives and old women,
> whose advice he would rather follow than theirs.[2]

When he died, his sister, Mary Turbeville, practiced in London "with good reputation and success."[3]

*The Ladies Dispensatory*, published in 1651, was written for the laywoman practitioner. Women took private coaching in medicine as all medical schools were closed to them. As Sarah Fell noted in her accounts:

> July ye 5 1674 by Mo to Bro: Lower yt hee gave Thomas Lawson
> for comeinge over hither to Instruct him & sisters, in the knowl-
> edge of herbs 10.00.[4]

The care of the sick and the poor was considered to be the duty of a person of quality, and housekeepers were expected to have a competent knowledge of "phisick and chirurgery." The provision made by Lady Falkland of "antidotes against infection and of Cordials . . . of her Neighbours as should need them, amounted yearly to very considerable summes . . . her skill indeed was more than ordinary."[5]

Elizabeth Bedell "was very famous and expert in Chirurgery, which she continually practiced upon multitudes that flock'd to her, and still gratis, without respect of persons, poor or rich."[6]

Entries in the diaries of the times show how expert women were in the art of healing. One entry by the Reverend Josselin reads: "my Lady was my nurse & Phisitian & I hope for much good. . . . I took purge & other things for it."[7]

Marmaduke Rawdon had a carriage accident and strained his arm, "but comminge to Hodsden his good cossen Mrs Williams, with hir arte and care, quickly cured itt, and in ten dayes was well againe."[8]

## Elizabeth Countess of Kent

Elizabeth Countess of Kent was famous for her obstetric and medical skills. She wrote *Manual of Choice Remedies* or *Rare Secrets in Physic and Surgery,* which was published in 1670. It was a bestseller and by 1687 had gone into nineteen editions, a sign of the public interest in all aspects of medicine and how it was still seen to be a popular skill, which many people wanted to learn.

## Oliva Sabuco des Nantes Barrera

Oliva Sabuco des Nantes Barrera (b. 1562) was author of a number of philosophical books on the nature of humanity and the workings of the human body. She speculated as to the cause of the plague and believed it was due to an airborne poison which attacked the brain, causing the body to lose too much heat and moisture and thus disturbing the body's equilibrium. She discussed the effect of pain on people and how fear and other emotional states affected the body. Her psychological theories were far in advance of her time, and she incurred the wrath of the inquisitors who ordered her books destroyed. Only two copies of her original works remain, and both of these are badly defaced. Her first book, however, was published again in the seventeenth century. Written in Spanish, it considers humanity in relation to the world, health, old age, and certain political and social reforms.[9] Clearly Oliva Sabuco was an advanced thinker, but as only fragments of her work remain, we cannot tell very clearly what her concerns were.

## Sophia of Mechlenburg

Sophia was the mother of Christian IV of Denmark and Norway. When her son was born, she refused to have the usual medical men present and allowed only a midwife and a nurse to be in attendance. She insisted on feeding the child herself, which was unheard of in those days. She encouraged women in Scandinavia to breastfeed and to use birth control and demanded that midwives be thoroughly trained in and taught the basic rules of hygiene. Cleanliness was not practiced at the time, but Sophia's vigorous public campaign paid off. (To this day Denmark has one of the lowest infant mortality rates in the world.)

Sophia advocated the isolation of those who had infectious diseases, the use of exercise, and the benefits of a healthy diet in combating illness and introduced the fumigation of clothes in cases of pestilence. She made sure that burials were carried out more effectively and launched a campaign to stop the infanticide of illegitimate babies. She also encouraged her subjects to bathe more regularly and to kill body lice. As a result, public health in general improved and the mortality rate declined during her regency. A pioneer in public health measures, she also made laws relating to the proper burial of bodies and public health education.

## Margarita Fuss

Margarita Fuss (b. 1555) was the daughter of a noblewoman *accoucheuse* (birth attendant) who was forced to earn her living after her husband proved incapable of organizing his finances. She studied medicine, initially with her mother, and then went to Strasbourg and Cologne for further education. She became famous and in such demand that she traveled all over Germany, Holland, and Denmark delivering babies. Known as "Mother Greta," she had a unique style. She dressed in a red-and-black striped skirt, a jacket like that worn by Hungarian hussars, and in winter a cape trimmed with yellow fur and carried a bag with a snake emblem embroidered on it and a gold-headed cane.

Margarita died in 1626 having been appointed court physician and midwife. The cathedral bells were rung in her honor to commemorate her life and work.

In the seventeenth century, women were increasingly squeezed out of public life and they retreated into midwifery and nursing, the only areas of medicine considered suitable for their "lowly" skills, although even these areas were no longer exclusively the domain of women.

Traditionally, midwifery had been one area in which women had had some power, though even this area of medicine was not sacrosanct for women. Midwives were able to earn a lot of money, so economically it made sense for men to attempt to usurp this field. One famous midwife, Hester Shaw of Barking, was said to have been paid £1000 for delivering a son to a Mrs. Perrot in August 1666. The only training for those wishing to study midwifery was by apprenticeship. Many midwives gained their skills solely by observation. In rural England it was customary, when a woman started in labor, to send for the neighbors, partly to bear witness to the child's birth and partly to spread the knowledge of midwifery, because in an emergency any woman might be called on to minister to the mother and baby. Several handbooks were written with this in mind, such as Jane Sharp's *The Midwives Book*. It was the result of thirty years in practice. She wrote the book using simple language on purpose, so that it might be accessible to the most humble of midwives. Jane Sharp insisted that midwives should have an understanding of how the human body worked before practicing. Her book included anatomy, the signs of pregnancy, postpartum disease, how to choose a nurse, and how to care for a baby. She wrote that she had

> often sate down sad in the Consideration of the many Miseries Women endure in the Hands of unskilful Midwives; many professing the Art without any skill in anatomy, which is the Principal part.

She said that midwives must be both speculative and practical, and says that midwifery is

> the natural propriety of women. . . . It is not hard words that perform the work, as if none understood the Art that cannot understand Greek. Words are but the shell, that we oftimes break our Teeth with them. . . . It is commendable for men to employ their spare time in some things of deeper Speculation than is required of the female sex; but the art of midwifery chiefly concerns us.[10]

Nicholas Culpeper (1616–1654), a famous herbalist of the seventeenth century, also wrote a book for midwives, which became a bestseller. He was almost the only male medic who thoroughly disapproved of male midwives, as is shown by the following quote:

> worthy Matrons, You are of the number of those who my soul

loveth, and of whom I make daily mention in my Prayers. . . . If you please to make experience of my rules, they are very plain, and easie enough. . . . If you make use of them, you wil find your work easie, you need not call for the help of a Man-Midwife, which is a disparagement, not only to yourselves, but also to your Profession . . . All the Perfections that can be in a Woman, ought to be in a Midwife. . . . If *any want Wisdom, let him ask it of God,* not of the colledg of Physitians, for if they do, they may hap go without their Errand, unless they bring Money with them. [11]

## Elizabeth Cellier

Elizabeth Cellier tried to organize the profession for both study and work. At the time (1642) midwives were licensed by the Chirurgion's Hall, but not before they had passed three examinations before six midwives and six surgeons skillful in the art. By 1662 this practice had stopped, by which time the process was reduced to paying a fee to the Doctors' Commons and taking an oath against the papacy. With the relaxing of the rules of examination the levels of infant mortality increased. Cellier petitioned James II in 1687 to unite midwives by a Royal Charter. She presented him with the following figures: in the twenty years from 1642 to 1662, 6000 Englishwomen had died in childbirth, that is, 300 per year. There were also an estimated 13,000 miscarriages and 5000 newborn deaths, which, she claimed, were preventable. Cellier maintained that the vast majority of these deaths were due to the unskilled nature of birth attendants. She proposed a royal maternity hospital, staffed by trained birth attendants, to be a model of cleanliness and neatness, and suggested that in this hospital they might also train midwives and nurses and provide homes for illegitimate babies. Cellier outlined her plans in detail in an attempt to raise the required amount of money, but this came to nothing owing to timidity on the part of her colleagues and public apathy. She persisted, however, and put her plans before the king. He refused to support her plans and, outraged, she spoke out publicly against the monarchy and was put in the stocks for her troubles and forced to watch her books being burnt before her eyes.[12]

Cellier proposed that midwives of the first rank should be limited in numbers to 1000 and that they should pay a fee of £5 on admittance to the guild and the same amount should be paid annually. All midwives of this rank should be eligible for the position of matron or assistant to the government. Other midwives should be admitted to the second thousand on payment of half that sum. The money from these fees was to be used to erect "one good large and convenient house or hospital for the receiving and taking in of exposed children, to be subject to the care, conduct and management of one governess, one female secretary, and twelve matron assistants . . . the children afterwards educated to their several capacities." Cellier also proposed that collecting boxes be placed in every church, chapel, or public place of divine service and that the hospital be allowed to establish twelve lesser hospitals in twelve of the larger parishes, each to be governed by twelve matrons, assistants to the corporation of midwives for women to give birth and to rest after childbirth. The king united midwives by Royal Charter, but he would do no more.

Noblewomen had relative freedom and also the means by which to study. One such, Lady Willoughby, went to Italy to study medicine. She was called to practice after the death of her baby and those of her three neighbors. She collected herbs and studied their medicinal properties and after returning from her studies set up in practice. Other noble ladies who were known to practice medicine include: Lady Warwick, Lady Alice Lucy, Lady Mainard, and Lady Arundell who wrote a book called *Physick and Chirgery*. Lady Mainard, living during the time of Charles II of England, was said to be "the common physician of her sick neighbours. . . . [S]he would dress their loathsome sores, give them diet and lodging until they were cured, and bury them if they died."[13]

Anne Woolley of London wrote a book on diet and medicine for women in 1674. Even more adventurous was Lady Anne Halkett (1622–1699) who served as a surgeon in the Royal Army at the battle of Dunfermline. At Perth in 1650, after the battle of Dunbar, she was personally thanked by the king. As well as surgeon she was also nurse, midwife, and physician. She was captured and held prisoner in Newcastle where she was called upon to treat the inmates and deliver babies. She was believed to have helped the King of Scotland, James II, to escape his enemies disguised as a woman. In gratitude he gave her an award of £100 per year.

## Louyse Bourgoise

Louyse (or Loyse) Bourgoise (1563–1636) was a famous French midwife. She studied in the Parisian suburb of Saint Germain. She later married Martin Boursier who was assistant to the famous surgeon Ambroise Pare. When Henry II sacked the suburbs in 1590, she was forced to flee with her three children and her mother. She learned midwifery from Pare and her husband, and when peace was restored, she joined the guild of midwives and began to practice. She became midwife to the nobility and by 1609 had attended two thousand births. Her first major treatise was published in 1609.[14] It was the most comprehensive work on obstetrics since Trotula's work, written many centuries previously. She covered anatomy, diagnosis, the stages of pregnancy, abnormalities of labor and directions in which to turn the fetus, multiple births, postnatal care, and breast-feeding. Recognizing that poor nutrition was a factor in anemia, she was the first to suggest adolescent girls should be given iron supplements, thus treating the cause and not the symptoms. The second edition of this book, published in 1617, included a long list of clinical cases. It went through many revised editions and was translated into four languages. The author warned that syphilis, the scourge of Europe, could cause sterility and contaminate the fetus, resulting in the death of the newborn.

## Angelique-Marie Leboursier Ducoudray

Madame Angelique-Marie Leboursier Ducoudray (1712–1789) was for twenty-two years professor of obstetrics and anatomy in France. She developed the use of anatomical models to teach delivery techniques and published a text book in 1759, which went into five editions. And in 1759, despite vehement opposition from male surgeons, she was awarded an annual stipend by Louis XV to teach obstetrics in hospitals throughout France.

At this time the Americas were being colonized by Europeans, many of them having fled from political and religious persecution at home. Women were acting as midwives, nurses, physicians, and surgeons. In Quebec in 1664, Jeanne Mace (1603–1673) opened a hospital, probably the first of its kind, in what was later to become Canada. These pioneering women had, through necessity, a freedom denied them in Europe. With populations so small and scattered, anyone, regardless of sex, who could doctor was warmly welcomed. It is to be assumed that these colonizers learned about local plants from Native American women. Little acknowledgment, however, is given to this interchange. The gifts the Europeans brought were often of less value. They were responsible for spreading smallpox, venereal disease, measles, and influenza. These colonizers were hardy women; Mrs. Thomas of Marlborough was said to have traveled up to her eighty-seventh year on horseback or on snowshoes through hundreds of miles of forest, caring for mothers and their babies. A Mrs. Whitmore of Vermont is remembered by her tombstone which says she officiated at over two thousand births and never lost one child—an astonishing record and the envy of any modern obstetrician.[15]

Women physicians were more numerous in Germany than in other European countries at this time. Eleanora, Duchess of Troppau, published six books on medicine. They had an enormous circulation and remained in print for over a hundred years. Some of her prescriptions are still in use today. One remedy for the Queen of Hungary is a salve for boils and abscesses, which used blackberry leaves, rosemary, and thirty other ingredients.[16]

## Maria Schürmann

A talented Dutch woman, Maria Schürmann (1607–1678) graduated in law from the University of Utrecht where she became a teacher of philology and history. She studied medicine and was especially interested in the treatment of eye diseases and blindness. She spoke twelve languages and read and wrote books in Latin, Arabic, and Hebrew on medical topics. She practiced as a physician and tended the sick at home and in hospitals. She was also an artist and a poet and a strong defender of women's rights. She refused to marry a Dutch poet named Cats so that she could devote all her attention to her work. In 1648 she wrote a thesis, demonstrating that intelligence was not a matter of gender.[17]

## Ellena Cornero

In Italy Ellena Cornero (1646–1684) was a linguist and scientist, famous throughout Europe. A native of Venice, she was a magistra of liberal arts in Padua and became a teacher there. A contemporary said of her that all the scholars of Rome and Siena sat at her feet. She lectured in mathematics and medicine and published a three-volume work in 1688.[18]

## Christina

Christina, daughter of the Swedish king, Gustavus Adolphus, was an avid scholar and learned woman. She studied astronomy, geology, and chemistry, and working with Descartes and Conring, she learned physics and history. She read all the Latin classics. Particularly interested in pharmacology, she did a great deal of research into chemistry and its application to medical science. She corresponded with the great thinkers of her time and encouraged them to share their ideas. The Swedish court became filled with the most brilliant minds of the times. However, she was unpopular in Protestant Sweden for converting to Catholicism. She refused to marry, which was unheard of for a royal princess, and was openly a lesbian and dressed in men's clothes.[19] She shocked society wherever she went and was punished for this in later life. She spent a great deal of her country's money. Because of her unpopularity she abdicated the throne and traveled to Rome in 1654 where she continued to study chemistry and medicine. Twice she tried to regain her throne, but was unsuccessful both times. Her life was an enigma and she died alone and in poverty, having been abandoned by those she had known. She was remembered only by the pope who had a statue built in honor of her conversion.[20]

## The Countess of Chinchon

The Countess of Chinchon, wife to the Spanish viceroy to Peru, was credited with bringing the chinchona bark (quinine) to Europe. Sick and near death with malaria, the viceroy turned to the Peruvian Indians who journeyed far into the Andes to search out this bark. In 1638 she brought it home with her to Spain where there was a malaria epidemic. Linnaeus, the Swedish botanist, named it chinchona in her honor.

## Lady Montagu

Lady Montagu is credited with discovering a vaccination for smallpox. This disease was one of the great scourges of the seventeenth century, when the mortality rate for the disease was 50 percent. There were sixty thousand deaths in one year alone. Louis XV of France and Mary Queen of England both died from the disease, which was no respecter of rank or privilege. Lady Montagu noticed that Turkish women inoculated their children against the disease. In 1717 she wrote the following in a letter to a friend:

> The smallpox, so fatal, and so general among us, is here entirely harmless by the invention of ingrafting, which is the term they give it. There is a set of old women who make it their business to perform the operation every autumn in the month of September when the great heat is abated . . . the old woman comes with a nutshell full of the matter of the best sort of smallpox.[21]

A vein was opened and a little of the venom put into the opening and the hollow shell bound over the wound. The patient had a slight fever for two days but no pitting. "The pus was taken from a healthy child on the thirteenth day . . . and carried on from patient to patient."[22] It became the fashion for the rich to thus inoculate themselves against this dreaded disease despite vehement opposition from the medical profession and the church.

## Elizabeth Blackwell

In the eighteenth century Elizabeth Blackwell (1712–1770) wrote *The Curious Herbal,* published in 1737. She was a physician and obstetrician. She studied botany and anatomy with her husband who was an apothecary, and with Dr. James Douglas who was a famous obstetrician and surgeon. Her husband was jailed for debt in 1737, and Blackwell's book paid his fine. An unlucky man, he was eventually executed for conspiracy against the king of Sweden. *The Curious Herbal,* beautifully illustrated with five hundred copper-engraved drawings, is in two volumes. The specimens were taken from the physic garden in Chelsea, which was then owned by Sir Hans Sloane who became a friend of hers. Blackwell later studied obstetrics with Dr. Smellie, a well-respected doctor, and eventually established a highly successful practice of her own.

## Martha Mears

Martha Mears wrote *The Pupil of Nature, or Candid Advice to the Fair Sex* in 1797, a book on gynecology and obstetrics that went into five editions. She described the use of forceps, discussed measures to avoid childbed fever, and advised on general hygiene. She saw pregnancy as a natural event and not something needing to be controlled or as a medical emergency. Martha Mears encouraged pregnant women to love the arts and to commune with nature. She encouraged and enabled women to study at the new lying-in hospitals alongside men, a great breakthrough for her time.

## Mrs. Hutton

Mrs. Hutton was a famous woman herbalist who pioneered the use of digitalis or foxglove. The Dean of Oxford was brought to her door

dying from congestive heart disease. She cured him and became famous overnight. Dr. Withering heard of this cure and after much
bartering with her bought the recipe. Hutton had discovered that the
plant had to be picked at certain times and be used in combination
with other remedies to temper its effect. She was a botanist and
pharmacist who experimented with dosages and various mixtures,
preparing the remedy in many forms to make the best use of it. She
was not, as medical history would have us believe, an old wife who just
happened upon this plant, but a trained and thoughtful practitioner
who had used the herb on patients, monitored its effects, and perfected a mixture for congestive heart failure and water retention. We
do not know how she came to sell the remedy to Dr. Withering or how
much money he offered her; we know only that it passed into the
British Pharmacopea under his name in 1785 and that it is used to this
day for heart failure.

## Salomee Anne Roussietski

Salomee Anne Roussietski (b. 1718) was married at age thirteen to
Halpir, an occultist who took her to Constantinople where he had a
medical practice. She studied medicine with him, and they worked
together. In a very short space of time, she became more successful
than him. He was jealous and angry and one day ran off with all the
money, leaving her penniless with her newborn baby. After recovering
from the birth, and presumably from the shock, she borrowed money
from some wealthy Turks and moved to Adrianople and then to other
cities, earning her living by practicing medicine. She found Halpir in
Sophia, sick and penniless himself, and took pity on him, nursing him
back to health. But shortly thereafter he contracted the plague and
died. Alone again, she was pressured by a wealthy Turk to marry him,
but she was not interested. He was so angry that he had her arrested
as a spy. While she was in jail, she cured the jailer of erysipelas and he
helped her to escape. She eventually arrived back in her hometown,
started up another practice, and married again. When the Austrian–
Turkish war broke out, she traveled to Petersburg to liberate some of
her friends, but when she returned she found that her second husband

had absconded with the funds and that she was pregnant again. She built up yet another practice and in 1759 returned to Constantinople, eventually becoming physician to the Harem of Moustapha, where presumably she was safe from men. What happened to her after this is unknown.

Three countries, Turkey, Austria, and Poland, claim Salomee Anne Roussietski as their first medical woman.

# 8

# *W*omen Enter the Profession: The Struggles of Nineteenth–Century Women Doctors

*I had no medical companionship, the profession stood aloof, and society was distrustful of the innovation. Insolent letters came by post, and my pecuniary position was a source of constant anxiety.*

Elizabeth Blackwell
*on her experiences as the first medical woman* [1]

THE RISE OF THE SUFFRAGETTE MOVEMENT IN THE UNITED STATES and Europe heralded campaigns for women to enter the professions and to participate in the professional life of their countries. Gradually universities opened their doors to women students, and the idea of the middle-class professional woman began to gain public acceptance, if not approval. Medicine was one of the last male bastions to be besieged by women, and their fight to be allowed to study medicine was long and bitter. Although by this time it was neither possible nor expedient to burn women healers at the stake, the physical and psychological violence these pioneering women underwent at times resembled torture in an inquisitor's cell.

Wealthy middle- and upper-class women in Europe and the United States struggled to gain acceptance into medical schools. Some were

committed radicals, like Sophia Jex-Blake, while others were as politically backward as their male colleagues. Elizabeth Garrett-Anderson,
for instance, was anxious that the "wrong" kind of woman should not
be admitted to medical training for women. Presumably this meant
from the wrong class or race, or from a radical or political background.

Some of the new women doctors embraced the popular health
movements of the nineteenth century (nature cure, hygiene, and preventive medicine), while others were fearful of inviting further ridicule from the male medical profession and urged their women colleagues to observe orthodox scientific doctrine and not to follow any
new medical treatments.

## Harriot Hunt

Harriot Hunt (1805–1875) is widely recognized as the first qualified
practitioner, although there was no general registering body for doctors in the United States at that time. She was inspired to practice
medicine because of her sister's long illness, which did not respond to
traditional treatments. Her sister was finally cured by an herbalist,
Mrs. Mott, and both Hunt and her sister decided to study with her.
After Hunt's training, she set up practice in Boston in 1835. She
describes bitterly her experience of being a lone practitioner: "If I had
cholera, hydrophobia, smallpox or any malignant disease, I could not
have been more avoided than I was."[2] She was ostracized by her male
colleagues and denied access to medical institutions for fear that
women would be a distraction to male students. After twelve years in
practice she decided to go for further medical training and applied to
Harvard Medical School. She sent her application to Oliver Wendell
Holmes, Dean of the School, who was in favor of her application. It
was to no avail, however. At the time of her application, Hunt was
forty-two years old. A photograph shows her as a matronly figure,
unlikely to stir the sexual feelings of the younger male students.[3] Her
application was turned down as "inexpedient." She was outraged at
their meanness and unwillingness to review or even discuss their
decision. Previously Hunt had not been involved in any feminist

movements, but her unjust treatment politicized her, and she became a mainstay of the then burgeoning U.S. women's movement. When Hunt heard that Elizabeth Blackwell had been accepted at regular medical college, she resubmitted her application. This time she won the faculty over, which agreed to let her and three black men join the school. In her letter Hunt argued: "In opening your doors to women, it is mind that will enter the lecture room,"[4] clearly a reference to the fact that the four were medical students first and black and female second.

The other medical students, however, had different ideas. They claimed that if black men were allowed to enroll in the course it would lower the value of their degrees. They further claimed that Hunt was unsexing herself and must be banned to preserve the dignity of the school[5] and that the presence of black students was socially repulsive. None of the four was allowed to attend a single lecture. (The trustees of Harvard finally allowed women into medical school, almost a hundred years later in 1944.)

Hunt continued to practice medicine and after twenty-five years received an honorary medical degree from the Female Medical College of Pennsylvania in 1853.

Like many women practitoners, she was interested in preventive medicine. In her practice, she concentrated on diet, exercise, and healthy clothing. The fashions of her day were extremely uncomfortable, at times dangerous to health. Women narrowed their waists by tight, suffocating corsets, and sometimes had their ribs broken or removed to make their waists still smaller. In addition, their bodies had to bear the weight of heavy crinolines and the supporting framework with its many layered petticoats.

Hunt believed that many illnesses were social or had a psychological basis, and for these reasons she maintained that women doctors had a clear advantage over men, as they were more sympathetic and better listeners. As part of her work, she gave hundreds of lectures to women's groups on women's health as part of her drive to educate the lay public about their bodies and their functions. She remained determined to "awaken public thought to the positive need of women entering the profession."[6]

On the silver anniversary of her practice, her friends crowned her with flowers and gave her a gold ring to honor her marriage to the profession. When she died in 1875, she was buried under a statue of Hygeia, goddess of healing, commissioned from a black woman sculptor, Edmonia Lewis.

## Elizabeth Blackwell

If Hunt was seen as the United States' first medical professional, Elizabeth Blackwell (1821–1910) was its first medical student. She was born in England, in Bristol, into a nonconformist family. Her father, Samuel Blackwell, was a follower of Wilberforce, the antislave campaigner. Blackwell was politicized at an early age and recalls how she and her sister gave up eating sugar as a protest against the slave trade. Her family emigrated to the United States in 1832, settling in Cincinnati. After her father's death, Blackwell and her sister ran a school to support the family and she became involved in the struggle for education for women. In 1845 she decided to embark on a medical career after seeing a friend die, having declared her friend would not have suffered as much had she been attended by a woman. She naturally received no encouragement from the male doctors she contacted, but this only strengthened her resolve. "The idea of winning a doctor's degree gradually assumed the aspect of a great moral struggle, and the moral fight possessed immense attraction for me."[7] She described a conversation with a physician who tried to persuade her to give up her ambitions: "I told the doctor that if the path of duty led me to hell I would go there; and I did not think that by being with devils I should become a devil myself—at which the good Doctor stared."[8]

Blackwell approached a number of medical colleges. Although many were sympathetic to her in private, none would run the risk of public scandal or the wrath of the medical profession to take her on as a student. She was advised either to go to Paris to study or to enter medical school disguised as a man, but she replied: "It was to my mind a moral crusade on which I had entered, a course of justice and common sense, and it must be pursued in the light of day, and with public sanction, in order to accomplish its end."[9] Finally Geneva

Medical College in New York invited her to enroll. Although she was teased a little by the students, as a minority of one she did not represent a threat and therefore was both tolerated and patronized:

> . . . the ladies stopped to stare at me, as at a curious animal. I afterwards found that I had so shocked Geneva propriety that the theory was fully established either that I was a bad woman, whose designs would gradually become evident, or that, being insane, an outbreak of insanity would soon be apparent.[10]

She recalls her horror at witnessing how brutally male doctors treated female gynecological examinations: "It was a horrible exposure, indecent for any woman to be subjected to such a torture."[11] This experience and her internship at the women's syphilitic department of the Blockley Almshouse strengthened her resolve to qualify as a doctor so that women would have the opportunity to be treated by a member of their own sex.

Blackwell graduated in 1849 and traveled to England where she was well received. She was given permission to study on the wards of St. Bartholomew's and was welcomed by all the medical professors—with the exception of the professor for the diseases of women. Blackwell also met Florence Nightingale, and the two became lifelong friends, lending each other support and encouragement in their struggles to be accepted as health professionals.

When she returned to New York she opened a practice in an apartment there but found it hard going to make ends meet. There was a vast amount of opposition to her practicing, both within and without the medical profession. She faced persistent verbal and physical abuse from men who would wake her up in the middle of the night. Financial worries compounded her problems. "It is hard, with no support but a high purpose, to live against every species of social opposition. . . . I *should* like a little fun now and then. Life is altogether too sober."[12]

Like Harriot Hunt, Blackwell realized the importance of public education and in 1852 gave a series of lectures on physical education for girls. These proved to be very popular and were well attended. She had them printed up in a pamphlet and called them "Laws of Life in Relation to the Physical Education of Girls."

In 1853 she founded a small dispensary for working-class women and their children, which later became the New York Infirmary for Women and Children. It had a female resident medical staff and a male consulting board. Naturally it faced widespread opposition and terrible financial problems, but it was kept open with the support of local women's activists. It also provided a training ground for the new generation of medical students who followed in Blackwell's footsteps and was a way into practice for those women who qualified. Despite doubts that such an institution might increase the isolation of medical women, Blackwell decided to open a medical college for women in 1868. She added natural medicine in the curriculum, and she herself was in charge of the department of hygiene.

Blackwell returned to Europe. She delivered a series of lectures in Paris and submitted her name to be included on the lists of the General Medical Council and was accepted in 1859. She was the first and only woman to be registered until Elizabeth Garret-Anderson was admitted seven years later. In the same year, Blackwell went on a lecture tour throughout Great Britain and was involved in the fund-raising campaign to open a hospital for the treatment of the diseases of women and children.

Blackwell went back to New York and continued in private practice until 1869, when she decided to return to England and settle there permanently. She immediately became involved in the campaign against the Contagious Diseases Act, fired by what she had seen on the wards in New York—young servant girls dying of syphilis after having been seduced (raped) by their masters. The campaign was aimed at removing this act from the statute book. The act allowed for the state registration of prostitution under which women in certain areas might randomly be labeled as common prostitutes and forced to undergo periodic medical examination with the threat of prison should they refuse. The act was passed in 1864. This provided a lucrative salary for doctors, the union of doctors, and the state in a particularly sinister fashion. The women's campaign against the act stressed the violatory nature of the forced physical examination by the male doctors and the need for and importance of having trained women doctors who could perform these examinations. The medical profession was generally seen to be in support of the act as it provided an increase in status for its members. Blackwell continued working in the campaign until it was repealed seventeen years later. She set up private practice in London and was appointed to the chair of gynecology at the London School for Medical Women in 1874.

In her autobiography, Blackwell discusses her doubts about contemporary medical practice, including cautery (the burning of flesh that is diseased) and the use of mercury and other potentially toxic drugs. She had a strong Christian belief, and her spiritual values influenced her approach to the treatment of illness. Like her friend Florence Nightingale, she believed ethics and spiritual values had to influence medical practice. She saw disease as being the result of a state of moral, physical, and emotional imbalance and said she realized that the mind could not be separated from the body.[13] She was a firm believer in the value of preventive medicine through hygiene, diet, and sanitation. This theme is repeated over and over again in the lives of medical women, using the gentle, healing approach to medicine, rather than surgery or drastic remedies.

## Maria Zakrzewska

Maria Zakrzewska (1829–1902) was born in Berlin, the daughter of a Prussian army officer and midwife mother. She studied midwifery in a school in Prussia, La Charité, and in 1852 became its chief midwife. She was responsible for two hundred students, but finally resigned as she faced increasing hostility from the male medical professionals. She left for New York in 1853, but because of difficulties with the language, she found it impossible to gain employment and was forced to work in the manufacturing industry. In 1854 she returned to school, enrolling in the Cleveland Medical School in Ohio. She faced great opposition and social pressure as a student and found it extremely hard even to find a place to stay. Her fees at Ohio were paid by Harriot Hunt who had been fund-raising for this very purpose. This was a lifesaver for Zakrzewska whose business venture had by this time all but collapsed.

Carol Severence, head of the local physiological society, paid for her lodgings. When she graduated in 1856 she could not find premises to practice in as the male landlords did not believe that she intended to start a clinic and thought that it was a front for something else. They didn't think she would earn enough money to pay the rent. She finally set up her practice in Elizabeth Blackwell's back parlor. She found it very hard to find patients, as there were few established women's networks, and the general public had little confidence in the abilities of women physicians.

Unlike Hunt and Blackwell, Zakrzewska was in agreement with establishment medicine and against any form of alternative treatment or anything which might be construed as a threat to the medical status quo. She recognized the power of the medical establishment and was unwilling to take up any position which might jeopardize her career.

In 1859 she moved to Boston and was appointed professor of obstetrics and the diseases of women and children at Samuel Gregory's Female Medical College. But in 1862 she resigned from the college after quarreling with Gregory and founded the New England Hospital for Women and Children. Women activists in Boston supported this venture by raising funds for the hospital, staffing it, and providing a network for finding patients. They also provided the emotional and moral support that Zakrzewska, as a pioneer, so badly needed. Naturally, it was hard going at the beginning, but the financial hardship was eased by the gifts and bequests which came flooding in. Over 80 percent of all donations were from women.

The New England's Women's Club was formed in 1869 and organized a support network for the hospital. The woman's journal also provided a mouthpiece for debates and gave publicity to the venture. The journal was outspoken in its attacks on male medicine's exclusion of women and the tactics used to intimidate and discourage women from studying and practicing medicine. It also gave free publicity to the hospital and to women doctors in the area, as the medical register of Boston refused to list female physicians practicing in the city.

The hospital specialized in obstetrics and gynecology as well as pediatrics. It also provided surgical facilities for these disciplines as well as a dispensary. It was extremely unusual that obstetrics and gynecology should be available under the same roof. The hospital had a fine record and became increasingly popular for women who wanted to have a safe delivery. At that time, huge numbers of women died in childbirth because of ignorance and bad practice by doctors.

In 1856 the Boston Lying-in Hospital was closed owing to an epidemic of puerperal fever (infection after childbirth), and women refused to go there any longer. The women also objected to the presence of male midwives and to the surgery that was performed on women, often unnecessarily. For example, female castration, or oophorectomy, was the fashion in the United States in the 1880s. J. Marion Sims (d. 1883) was known at the time as the "father of gynecology" and also, incredibly, as the "architect of the vagina." He was well known for his hatred and abhorrence of female organs.[14] He began his life's work performing dangerous gynecological surgery on black female slaves housed in a small building in his backyard. He then moved to the women's hospital in New York, performing these operations on women in front of an exclusively male audience. Mary Smith suffered thirty operations under his hands between 1856 and 1859; a black woman slave, Anarcha, suffered the same number ten years earlier in his backyard.

Mary Daly maintains: "For the next several decades ovariotomy became the gynecological craze; it was claimed to elevate the moral sense of the patients, making them tractable, orderly, industrious and cleanly."[15]

In 1848 Dr. Charles Meigs claimed that female organs exert "strange and secret influences" on "the very soul of woman."[16]

Dr. Ely van de Warker wrote in 1906 in defense of, and to protect, the ovary, but his reasoning reveals the reasons for his outrage.

> A woman's ovaries belong to the commonwealth; she is simply their custodian. Without them her life is stultified. Making a guess at figures . . . the one hundred and fifty thousand physicians of the United States have sterilized one hundred and fifty thousand women. Some of this large number have openly boasted, when the lunacy was at its height, that they have removed from fifteen hundred to two thousand ovaries. Assuming that each of

these women would have become the mother of three children, we have a direct loss of five hundred and fifty thousand for the first generation and one million six hundred and fifty thousand in the second generation.[17]

Zakrzewska's experience in La Charité stood her in good stead and gave her a solid grounding in hospital management. In 1889 the hospital published a report on 187 cases of midwifery practice, discussing asepsis and the debate about hygienic procedures. At that time, despite so-called medical advances, the aseptic procedures of Trotula and Hildegard had long been forgotten; it was not uncommon for doctors to go from the dissecting room, where they cut up diseased and infected dead bodies, to the delivery room, without even washing their hands. And at that time there were no rubber gloves. Women died in the tens of thousands owing to lack of care. But the medical profession was adamant in resisting the germ theory and the practice of commonsense hygienic procedures. Doctors did not believe that dirt and disease could be spread from one person to another through unclean hands, soiled bed linen, or dirty eating utensils. The Boston Lying-in Hospital closed three times in as many years due to outbreaks of puerperal fever. In contrast, the women's hospital in Boston grew and by the end of the century over nineteen hundred women had passed through its doors each year. Dr. Kate Campbell Hurd-Mead was interned at the hospital in the 1880s and reported that it was run efficiently on highly structured lines, yet was caring. By its twenty-fifth anniversary, it had become a women's hospital, staffed entirely by and for women.

Zakrzewska's own words sum up how she felt when she contemplated the busts of the famous men in Westminster Abbey, wondering if there would ever be a monument to the first woman physician:

> because she had the energy, will and talent . . . because she is a landmark of the era marked by women's freeing themselves from the bondage of prejudice and the belief that they are the lower being when compared to men . . . we need such landmarks of civilisation . . . because the now living, as well as those who will

live long afterward, need encouragement. . . . The person who is covered by a monument is of no consequence, but the fact that a "woman" can work and make an impression upon civilisation needs to be known and remembered.[18]

# Elizabeth Garrett-Anderson

In the United States women's struggle to become doctors was in many respects easier than in England. Doctors were far less organized and did not wield as much power. The English Medical Act of 1859 set up a General Medical Council to oversee education and to publish a list of qualified medical practitioners. It did not outlaw unqualified practioners but allowed licensing bodies to exclude women from their ranks should they choose to do so. Thus the early pioneer women who obtained medical degrees abroad were able to practice quite legally. The struggle for medical education and acceptance by the General Medical Council of women was a far more bitter and acrimonious experience for the women concerned, but once they won their victory, it was not open to challenge. The pioneer in the struggle was Elizabeth Garrett-Anderson.

She was born in 1836 to a wealthy businessman. She was sent to the academy for the daughters of gentlemen in Blackheath, and in 1854 she met Emily Davies through a school friend. Davies was a prominent member of the campaign for higher education for women in the 1860s and 1870s. In 1859 Garrett-Anderson attended Elizabeth Blackwell's lectures in London and was so inspired she decided to train as a doctor herself. Initially, her father was against the decision but was persuaded by the age-old argument that it was better that women be treated by women physicians, and also by the opposition his daughter encountered every step of the way.

Garrett-Anderson began by studying at Middlesex and was later allowed to attend ward rounds and to study with the apothecary. She approached Dr. Nunn of the dissecting room who allowed her to attend dissections when an assistant was present. Later that year, in 1860, she was allowed to attend Materia Medica lectures. Her problems began when she passed her examinations with distinction; the students successfully lobbied the lecturers to have her banned from the classes as it caused them "inconvenience." The *Lancet,* a medical journal, supported the banning, and in its edition of 1861 remarked: "The advance guard of the Amazonian army which has so often threatened our ranks, on paper, has already carried the outposts and entered the camp."[19] The bellicose nature of the editorial was a mere taste of the bloody battle to follow. Throughout their campaign, both the *Lancet* and the *British Medical Journal* remained extremely hostile and provided a mouthpiece and vociferous support for the medical establishment opposed to women's entry into the profession.

Garrett-Anderson then approached all the teaching hospitals in London and was rejected by each in turn. Finally, the Society of Apothecaries agreed to let her sit their examinations. Because no London university would let her attend lectures, she went to St. Andrew's, Scotland, where George Day, the Regius professor of medicine at the university, gave her private tuition and through his contacts and approval of her cause arranged for her to take private lessons from a variety of medical specialists. With the certificates of competence from these tutors, she applied to the Society of Apothecaries to be allowed to take their professional examinations. Well aware of the hornets' nest that this would stir up, they tried to back-pedal. But when Garrett-Anderson's father threatened legal action, they backed down, and she was able to take the final examinations. In October 1865, she became a Licentiate of the Society of Apothecaries, and in September of the following year, she was put on the medical register. Scared by the threat of an invasion by women, the apothecaries closed ranks and amended their rules so that only those who had attended medical school might take their exams. As all medical schools were closed to women, this meant only men could qualify.

Garrett-Anderson set up a private practice in London. As with all women practitioners, it was a struggle to make ends meet and to build up a sufficient caseload. However, slowly patients arrived, often more out of curiosity to see how she would treat them. Josephine Butler, a campaigner for women's rights and against the slave trade, was one:

> But for Miss Garrett I must say of her that I gained more from
> her than any other doctor; for she not only repeated exactly what

all the others had said, but entered much more into my mental
state and way of life than they could because I was able to tell her
so much more than I ever could or would tell any man.[20]

As Catriona Blake argues,[21] this clearly exposes the double threat that
women doctors have always posed to male medicine: first, that they
would take their patients away, but more importantly, that they would
provide an alternative to the new scientific worldview. That is, that
women listen and are sympathetic, and are more interested in the
mental-emotional aspects of disease as well as prevention and healing,
usually with noninterventionist and life-supporting therapies.

Garrett-Anderson opened the St. Marylebone Dispensary for
Women and Children in 1866. The dispensary was welcomed because
yet another outbreak of cholera had occurred in London in 1866.
Cholera, disease of poor sanitation, spread like wildfire through the
terrible slums of London. The local people welcomed any measure
that might reduce the risk of an epidemic. The large numbers of
women and children who attended the clinic indicated the desperate
need for medical services for the poor. At its inception, between sixty
and ninety women came each afternoon.

Garrett-Anderson, determined to gain her degree, then enrolled in
the Sorbonne. She passed the first examinations in March 1869, submitted her thesis in January 1870, and was awarded her medical
degree in June 1870. Her thesis was on migraines. She chose this topic
because it did not require her to use laboratory facilities to which she
would probably have been denied access. She discusses the treatment
of migraines from a holistic point of view, following the route of many
women practitioners. (She was against the increased specialization of
medicine.) She advocated a change of diet, fresh air, exercise, and no
alcohol, rather than any medication.

In 1870 she was given the honor of being the first woman doctor in
recent history to be awarded a medical post when she was appointed
visiting medical officer at the East London Hospital for Children. That
same year she was invited to stand as a candidate for the London
School Board elections and in May of that year was elected after
campaigning long and hard. One of the issues she worked on was the

education of girls. She insisted that girls should be taught only by women teachers.

In 1871 a committee was formed to raise funds for a new women's hospital in London, staffed by women doctors. They proposed to turn the room above the dispensary into a clinic. The dispensary had expanded rapidly; over 40,000 women had visited it in five years, even though patients had to pay a small fee while there was a free dispensary at the nearby hospital staffed by male doctors. Over the years, women came from further afield and the clinic began to specialize in gynecology and obstetrics. Generally, the public supported the clinic, but the medical profession remained hostile. Some doctors claimed that these women who had qualified overseas were taking a shortcut to gain status and to build up a practice.

The new hospital for women was opened in February 1872, three months after the appeal was launched. Garrett-Anderson was reluctantly persuaded to become part of the teaching staff at the school, and she took the chair in gynecology. Eventually she was elected dean of the hospital medical school and stayed in that post until 1903. She was finally elected as a member of the British Medical Association in 1874. She died in 1917.

## Sophia Jex-Blake

If Elizabeth Garrett-Anderson was an example of the decorous, ladylike approach in the battle for women doctors, then her contemporary, Sophia Jex-Blake, was the virago. Unlike Garrett-Anderson she chose not to marry, saying marriage and professional life were incompatible. She was a far more abrasive opponent, but then her struggle was very much harder than Garrett-Anderson's, who was the only woman student of her time and therefore a curiosity rather than a threat. By the time Jex-Blake entered the fray, the threat of women doctors was taken very seriously and vigorously opposed.

Sophia Jex-Blake was born in Hastings in 1840 into an evangelical family. Educated by governesses and at boarding school, she studied at Queen's College London and later accepted a teaching post there in mathematics. In 1862 she went to Edinburgh to continue her education and began to formulate her plans to follow a medical career. She corresponded with Garrett-Anderson about the possibility of studying medicine at Edinburgh. In 1865 she stayed with Dr. Lucy Sewall in Boston who was resident physician at the New England Hospital for Women and Children. She was encouraged by the way the women's community in Boston supported the medical women and may well have used this as a model for her later struggles in Britain. Jex-Blake became fascinated with medicine and stayed on with Sewall, helping her in the hospital. She returned to England with Sewall and persuaded her parents to allow her to study at the hospital. Later she transferred to Massachusetts General Hospital. She applied to study at Harvard but was turned down on the grounds that there were no facilities for women students. In 1868 she joined Elizabeth Blackwell and her sister, Emily, as they were setting up the women's college in New York. Her father died that year and for a time she returned to England to be with her mother.

Jex-Blake published an essay "Medicine as a Profession for Women," in an anthology produced by Josephine Butler on the women's movement. The book, *Women's Work and Women's Culture,* was published in 1869. In the essay she included a short history of women in medicine, showing that women physicians were not a new phenomenon but had their roots in history. She accused learned men of preventing women from having access to medical knowledge[22] and maintained that women doctors would increase the body of knowledge about women's health. There was great ignorance about the functions of a woman's body. At that time doctors claimed that a woman was less likely to conceive in the middle of her menstrual cycle, the opposite of what was in fact the case. Jex-Blake tried not to alienate the medical profession, but it was clear she had a fairly low opinion of male doctors.[23]

Josephine Butler wrote on her behalf to several universities about the possibility of her undergoing a medical training. One positive response came from David Masson, professor of English at Edinburgh, and Sir James Simpson, a famous surgeon who suggested she try for her degree in Edinburgh. London University was closed to her as the medical elite of London teaching hospitals ferociously blocked any move to allow women to study there.

Jex-Blake decided to try Edinburgh and enlisted the support of several men, among them Alexander Russell of the *Scotsman*, who gave her both personal and professional support through the pages of his newspaper. Professor George Balfour, dean of the medical school, agreed to allow her to attend some of the summer courses and to bring her case before the faculty. One of the governing bodies of the university, the university court, met and declared that although they were not opposed in principle to the idea of women students, they were not prepared to make special arrangements for one woman. This seemed a hopeful reply, despite the fact that 180 students petitioned that women should not be allowed in their courses as they claimed the material would have to be diluted for their consumption and that men's education would suffer as a result. An article in the feminist magazine the *English Woman's Review* in January 1870 hinted that Professor Christian, a staunch opponent to the cause, was behind the petition.[24] The medical profession through its journals was organizing a campaign of opposition to women and many of the arguments were based on the proposition that women would debase the profession and gradually lower standards.

Jex-Blake then applied to take the matriculation exams, (which meant she had to enroll at the university), and was accepted provided she organized separate lectures and found other women to join her in her studies. To this end she put an advertisement in *The Times* and received four replies: Isobel Thorne and Matilda Chaplin, who had both studied at the Female Medical College, Edith Pechey, who had an M.A. from Edinburgh, and Helen Evans. A year later Mary Anderson and Emily Bovel joined them, making it *septum contra Edinam* (seven against Edinburgh).

The original five were allowed to matriculate, and four were among the best seven of the 152 students. They were enrolled as medical students and became the first women undergraduates of a university in Great Britain. The women had to pay one hundred guineas for each class for the first year. Jex-Blake had the good fortune of being able to borrow the money from her mother to support those women who could not pay this substantial sum of money. There were also difficulties in finding enough lecturers for the classes, but they were rewarded by their dogged persistence. In the examinations four of the five women were in the honors list in chemistry and physiology, and all five won prizes in botany. Edith Pechey finished first in chemistry and should have been awarded the Hope Scholarship, consisting of money and, more importantly for her, access to the laboratories. But she was told she was not eligible, and the prize went to the man in second place. At the same time, the senate refused to issue the women with certificates for attendance to any of the classes.

The women appealed these unfair rulings, and the senate backed down over the issue of certificates, but not over the Hope Scholarship. The university came in for some heavy criticism over this decision, which was clearly not in the middle-class tradition of fair play. A satire in the *Daily Review* parodied the decision thus:

> . . . now it seems that the inferior sex are winning our scholarships over our most sacred heads. This is a matter which must be looked into. We will stand a great deal, but this is going too far; we must agitate. . . . We must have a bill for the protection of the superior sex.[25]

The adverse publicity hardened the opposition and heralded the beginning of the drive to exclude women entirely. The women continued to study, now in extramural classes, which gave them accreditation for the medical course. The male students then began a concerted campaign to intimidate and harass the women to give up their studies. A climax was reached on 18 November 1870 when the so-called Riot of Surgeons' Hall occurred.

As the women walked toward Surgeons' Hall, where they took their extramural classes, they encountered a drunken mob blocking the road. According to Jex-Blake, the crowd was large enough to block the traffic completely, but there was not a policeman in sight. When they reached the entrance, the gates were shut in their faces, and the mob pressing on them from behind meant they were in danger of being crushed. Fortunately, a student sympathetic to their cause saw what was happening, rushed out from the hall, and opened the gates to let the women through. The entire crowd poured into the courtyard and the women fled into their classroom. The howling, drunken mob continued to shout abuse throughout the class, and at one point a sheep was thrust through the door. When the class finished, they were escorted through the mob, who by now were screaming threats at them and throwing mud.

As a result of the riot, four students were reprimanded and fined, and the university threatened severe penalties should any student be brought before the magistrates. It was generally believed that the riot was incited by university professors. One male student sympathetic to the women wrote:

> May I venture to hint my belief that the real cause of the riots is the way some of the professors run you down in their lectures. They never lose a chance of stirring up hatred against you. For all I know they may have more knowledge of the riotous conspiracy than most people fancy.[26]

The women needed access to the infirmary to do their clinical training, but the infirmary board denied this. During one meeting, Jex-Blake made a speech in which she claimed that the rioters had been encouraged by the faculty and made allegations against Professor Christian's assistant, Mr. Craig. He then brought an action for damages against Jex-Blake. She lost the case and was fined a nominal farthing by the jury. The judge, however, overruled them and fined her the enormous sum of £915 11s 1d. Jex-Blake launched a public appeal to pay this, and in one month the fine was paid off.

The struggle continued as now even the extramural classes seemed in jeopardy, and the women were prevented from sitting the preliminary arts examination before the final degree course. The legal wrangles continued over whether the senate could give the women degrees and allow them to graduate. The Lord Ordinary, Lord Gifford, made a ruling that the university should recognize the extramural classes and allow the women to graduate. The university appealed his judgment and won. Costs were awarded against the women, far higher than the norm of £848. The women thus lost their four-year struggle to be allowed to graduate in medicine from a British university.

The physical and emotional toll on the women was hard. They were continually subjected to threats, sexual harassment, and obscene letters, while fighting legal battles, organizing defense committees and at the same time studying hard for their exams. Not surprisingly, it provided too great a task, and Jex-Blake failed her exams in 1872, adding to her already bitter defeat.

Jex-Blake went to Berne in Switzerland along with Edith Pechey to finish her studies. When they graduated, they both went to Dublin to take the examinations, which would finally allow them to have their names on the medical register. In 1877 a bill had gone through Parliament allowing foreign medical degrees to be recognized by the British medical registers. Passing their exams, Pechey and Jex-Blake became licentiates of King and Queen's College of Physicians of Ireland. Their names were finally entered on the medical register. Eliza Walker Dunbar and Louisa Atkins also graduated and joined Jex-Blake and Pechey on the British Medical Register.

The reaction of the medical profession was overwhelmingly hostile. The *Lancet* wrote on 17 August 1878:

> the law may recognise the qualifications obtained by women, but the profession must, in self respect, and we will not scruple to add in common decency, decline to accept them as titles of admission to the general body of practitioners. The confraternity of physicians and surgeons will not, we apprehend, either consult or hold professional intercourse with those who have assumed a position, and now desire to exercise functions, opposed to the instincts of their sex. Woman as nurse is the natural help of man. Woman as doctor is a conceit contrary to nature, and doomed to end in disappointment to both the physician and the sick.

Once qualified, Jex-Blake put herself up for the secretaryship of the London School of Medicine for Women, but failed to be elected. She then decided to move back up to Edinburgh where she set up in private practice. She soon had a thriving surgery as she was in great demand, the only woman practitioner in Scotland. In the first year she saw a total of 547 patients. In 1878 she opened a dispensary for poor women of the city. It was open two days a week and charged a small fee for medicines. Like the London clinic, it was soon full to bursting and saw over twenty-five hundred women in the first year. Larger premises were opened in 1885 with space for five beds. When she retired, she left her property in trust to open a hospital for women and children.

In 1886, Jex-Blake opened the Edinburgh School of Medicine for Women in Surgeons' Square. But she lacked the social skills to make it a success. Her dictatorial approach offended the students, and one of them went as far as to open a rival school for women. When Queen Margaret College opened in Glasgow and a medical course for women was started, Jex-Blake decided to close her school and became the first woman to lecture at the extramural school, teaching midwifery. She saw her years of campaigning come to fruition in 1894 when the University of Edinburgh finally opened its doors to women medical students, and the following year she was guest of honor at a ceremony celebrating the entry of women to the university medical colleges. In 1899 she retired to Sussex. Her written works included her graduation thesis on puerperal fever (1877), *The Care of Infants* (1884), and *Medical Women* (1886).

In its obituary of Sophia Jex-Blake, the *British Medical Journal* paid a belated tribute to the fighter who took on the medical establishment and won:

> Mentally Miss Jex-Blake was a woman of high ability and marked moral courage and determination. In addition she was possessed of many of the more commonly esteemed womanly qualities, though first and foremost, no doubt, she was an admirable fighter.[27]

## HOSPITALS FOR WOMEN RUN BY WOMEN

In November 1871 a series of lectures was published in *The Times* by Alice Westlake, treasurer of a committee established to found a women's hospital in London. She was appealing for funds. Many of the famous radicals of the day, including John Stuart Mill and the Earl of Shaftesbury, supported the project. They were planning to convert the rooms over the Marylebone dispensary into a temporary hospital while looking for premises that would have space for twenty beds. All the medical staff were to be women. The appeal was a success, and only three months after its launch, a hospital was opened in Seymour Place in February 1872. Elizabeth Garrett-Anderson performed surgery there and for twenty years was the only surgeon able to undertake the work. Given how successful the hospital was, she must have been sorely overworked. The hospital was a great success, despite the fact it had to charge a fee. In 1889 they moved to larger premises in Euston Road, £21,000 having been raised to pay for the new building. The prince of Wales laid the foundation stone. On her death, the hospital was renamed the Elizabeth Garrett-Anderson hospital.

After her retirement, Jex-Blake had left her clinic in trust for use should bed space be necessary. In 1900 enough funds had been raised to open the Edinburgh Hospital and Dispensary for Women and Children.

In 1912 Maud Chadburn started an appeal for another major hospital for women in South London. *The Times* inadvertently helped its cause by publishing a hostile letter. Immediately, £100,000 was donated, with the condition that the hospital be staffed only by women and that it treat women and children only. The South London Hospital for Women and Children was opened in 1914. Both the Elizabeth Garrett-Anderson and the South London provided vital training facilities, which allowed women medical students to graduate from London medical schools.

## THE LONDON SCHOOL OF MEDICINE FOR WOMEN

In 1874 Jex-Blake decided there was no alternative but to set up a medical school for women, all other points of entry into the profession having been closed to them. Jex-Blake spent the next two years working toward that goal and allowed her own studies to lapse.

A meeting was held in August of that year to establish a committee, and many influential people joined the movement. Jex-Blake became the secretary. In September a lease was signed on premises in Brunswick Square, and the school officially opened in October with fourteen students, twelve of whom had been studying in Edinburgh. To avoid accusations that their standards were lower than those of the men's colleges, the academic requirements were rigorous. Students had to take a preliminary examination and pay £200 for tuition, a large sum in those days. As yet there were no scholarships available.

They found their lecturers from among the already qualified medical women and from tutors at the men's medical colleges. The medical profession was uniformly hostile to the college and claimed it would never work and that any male staff member of a regular medical college who taught at the women's college was, by definition, second-rate and should be sacked. There was still no teaching hospital that would accept the women as students for clinical practice, neither would any of the nineteen examining bodies give the women the recognition they needed to be included in the medical register.

Elizabeth Garrett-Anderson and other medical women had disagreed in principle about the idea of separate education for women medical students. They saw it as a kind of educational apartheid, which would mean that women students would always be seen as second-rate. They were won over, however, by Jex-Blake's argument that they must appear united, at least in the public eye.

The personal and professional differences between Jex-Blake and Garrett-Anderson ran deep. Their style, their politics and ways of expressing themselves were very different. Garrett-Anderson was much more orthodox, a conservative who wanted women's entry into the profession but felt "the fair sex" should go about their fight quietly without making loud demands or being seen to be unwomanly. She was married to a respectable banker, and her experiences of studying did not have the trauma and bitterness of Jex-Blake's years at Edinburgh. She was the only woman studying at that time, and so was seen as an oddity, not part of an orchestrated campaign. Jex-Blake, on the other hand, was a firebrand and much in favor of confrontational politics. Her experiences at Edinburgh radicalized her and made her determined to change the system whatever the personal cost to herself. In her account of her struggle she wrote:

> We had begun to study simply because we saw no reason why women should not be the medical attendants of women. When we came in contact with such unexpected depths of moral grossness and brutality, we had burnt into our minds the strongest possible conviction that if such things were possible in the medical profession, women must, at any cost, force their way into it, for the sake of their sisters, who might otherwise be left at the mercy of such human brutes as these.[28]

The two women often disagreed about tactics and had several public arguments. Garrett-Anderson was at pains not to be seen as anti-man in any way and saw the movement for women doctors as simply allowing women to be on an equal footing with their male counterparts. She did not believe that women were necessarily better at treating women and claimed that women doctors could be wives and mothers, too; she herself had two children. Jex-Blake, on the other hand, said it was not possible to combine career and marriage. For the purposes of the school, however, the two women presented a united front, whatever their private misgivings.

The problem of clinical practice continued. The London Hospital at Whitechapel first agreed to allow women students but had to withdraw the offer when the male medical staff protested. Women could study at the hospital for women, but the medical examining bodies said it was too small to be accepted as a teaching hospital. In March 1877 the school struck a bargain with the managers of the Royal Free Hospital, allowing the women students access to its facilities in a five-year experiment. The managers were worried about the damage this might do to their reputation, and so the school had to compensate the hospital and medical staff for the possible fall-off in medical students. Enrollment at the school increased, however, and women students were able to receive a full medical education. An appeal was set up to find the money to pay the Royal Free fees.

In February 1878 the school was finally accepted by the secretary of state as one of the medical schools qualifying for the University of London examinations, and in September three women passed their examinations, which formed part of the medical degree at the university. In 1895 the London School of Medicine for Women wrote to the Royal College of Physicians and the Royal College of Surgeons asking to be admitted as there were, by that time, two hundred women on the register. Both colleges refused and it was not until 1910 that the joint board opened its examinations to women. The school continued to grow, however, and when its agreement with the Royal Free came up for review in 1882, it was automatically renewed at a greatly reduced fee. The experiment had proved to be a great success.

In 1883 the dean of the school resigned, and it was suggested that Garrett-Anderson be appointed. Jex-Blake traveled down from Edinburgh to oppose the motion and instead nominated Edith Pechey, but no one would second her. As hers was the only dissenting vote, Garret-Anderson was duly elected as dean, a post which she held until she retired in 1903.

By 1896 there were 159 students and they needed to expand the school. A fund was set up and by 1898 £12,000 had been raised. The new building was opened by the prince and princess of Wales. The acceptance of women doctors was almost complete and the school was renamed the London School of Medicine for Women. In 1900 it was officially recognized by the University of London.

## Mary Seacole

Mary Seacole presents us with the more familar face of a woman healer, an ordinary woman who pursued her art without pretense or fuss, simply concerned to heal suffering. She was born in Kingston, Jamaica, in 1805. Her mother was a healer, working in traditional medicine and with herbs. There was a strong tradition in Jamaica of doctors who treated wounds and performed surgery as well as treating internal diseases, and naturally they were the midwives. As Seacole said of herself: "I had from early youth a yearning for medical knowledge."[29]

As a child she experimented on herself and her pets to discover the effects of medicine. Her mother was married to a Scottish army officer and ran a boarding house in Kingston. Wounded officers came there to recuperate. She was a well-regarded healer who no doubt handed on much of her learning to her daughter.

Seacole married and traveled around the Caribbean and Central America. When her husband died, she returned to Kingston to run the boarding house. She was in the capital when the cholera outbreak of 1859 occurred, and her medical skills were in great demand. She treated some cases of the disease and was instructed by a Dr. B., who was living in her house, on how to manage the disease.

Later she set about traveling again, through Central America. While in Cruces there was a cholera epidemic about which she wrote:

> I believe that the faculty [of medicine] have not yet come to the conclusion that the cholera is contagious, and I am not presumptuous enough to forestall them; but my people have always considered it to be so.[30]

Again, like many women practitioners, she was well aware of the psychological component to physical illness: "It was scarcely surprising that the cholera should spread rapidly, for fear is its powerful auxillary."[31]

Such was her thirst for scientific knowledge that Seacole performed a postmortem on a child who died from cholera to find out more about the disease. In her treatment of the disease she used mustard plasters to raise local heat and emetics to purge and purify the body. The mustard plasters were applied to the spine and neck, and she took special care to keep the heart warm. She would give her patients cinnamon and water to drink. When the crisis was over, she would use strengthening medicines to avoid brain fever, which sometimes follows the acute phase of cholera. She had a holistic approach to medicine and believed that each case should be treated on its own individual merits.

> Few constitutions permitted the use of exactly similar remedies, and that the course of treatment which saved one man, would, if persisted in, have very likely killed his brother.[32]

When the Crimean War broke out in 1854, Seacole decided to offer her services to the troops at the front. She traveled to London and, once there, applied to the War Office to be a hospital nurse. She was familiar with the treatment of cholera, diarrhea, and dysentery, all of which were raging in the Crimea. But she was refused an interview. Undaunted, she applied to Elizabeth Herbert who was organizing the recruitment of nurses and was wife to the secretary of state for war, whom Seacole had been unable to see. But she got no more satisfaction from his wife than she did from the secretary of state. She was repeatedly denied an interview and, finally, after a long wait, was sent a message saying that no more nurses were needed. Clearly, being black was a factor in the doors being closed against her. Finally she spoke with one of Florence Nightingale's companions and subsequently made the remark: "I read in her face the fact, that had there been a vacancy, I should not have been chosen to fill it."[33]

Thwarted but undaunted by the narrow-minded prejudice and ignorance of the English middle class, Seacole decided to go under her own steam. She had cards printed which announced her arrival:

BRITISH HOTEL

Mrs. Mary Seacole

(Late of Kingston Jamaica)

Respectfully announces to her former kind friends

and to the officers of the Army and Navy generally,

That she has taken her passage in the screw steamer "Hollander,"

to start from London on the 25th of January,

intending on her arrival at Balaclava to establish a mess-table

and comfortable quarters for sick and convalescent officers.[34]

Seacole spent six weeks in Balaclava tending the sick and dying on the quayside. She worked alongside the army doctors, who were more than glad to have an extra pair of skilled hands. The wounded troops waited at Balaclava hospital to be transported to the base hospital at Scutari, four days' journey away. She baked cakes on a moored ship with eggs brought from Constantinople and wrote: "these with some lemonade, were all the doctors would allow me to give to the wounded.

They all liked the cake, poor fellows, better than anything else: perhaps because it tasted of 'home.'"[35]

She then opened a general store in Balaclava, selling supplies to the troops. It was an ambitious enterprise, the buildings and the yard cost £800 and took up an acre of space; it was later called the British Hotel. A poem in *Punch*, dated 6 December 1856, took up the story:

> she gave her aid to all who prayed
> To hungry and sick and cold:
> Open hand and heart, alike ready to part
> Kind words, and acts, and gold

Seacole provided both emotional and spiritual sustenance as well as good food and the company of women, reminding the men of the good things that they had left behind at home.

In 1855 when Sebastopol fell to the British, Seacole was the first woman there. In addition to running the hotel she traveled about with her bag of medicines, tending troops on the battlefield. After the assault on Redan, when there were enormous British casualties, she moved about the dead and dying, doing whatever she could to alleviate their suffering. In her book she writes: "Several times . . . I was ordered back, but each time my bag of bandages and comforts for the wounded proved my passport."[36]

She often gave her medicines and services free of charge; as a result, when the war ended and she returned to London, she faced economic disaster. By November 1856 she was in the bankruptcy courts. Letters from well-wishers responding to an appeal through *The Times* brought in enough money to pay her debts and enabled her to set up in business again. In July 1857 a grand military festival was held in her honor and over one thousand performers gave their services free. Unfortunately, little money was raised. Her fame merited editorials in *The Times*, for instance:

> I have seen her go down under fire, with her little store of creature comforts for our wounded men; and a more tender or skilful hand about a wound or broken limb could not be found among our best surgeons.[37]

No mention is made of Seacole in the writings about women's struggle to enter the medical profession. And this despite the fact that she was a skilled and practicing physician and surgeon. Clearly her color and class excluded her from the more rarified atmosphere of the salons where the ladies campaigning for medical education were to be found.

Her tale is a familiar one, the pioneering woman who feels called to practice medicine and follows the call despite enormous financial and personal hardship.

Her story ends well. Seacole spent the remaining years of her life traveling and working between London and Jamaica. She was awarded the Crimean Medal, the French Legion of Honour, and a Turkish medal. She acted as masseuse to the Princess of Wales, who was one of the patrons of her fund. She died in 1881 leaving a large fortune.

## James Barry

James Barry disguised herself as a man to study medicine at Edinburgh University and then joined the army as a doctor. She had a reputation because of her pioneering work in preventive medicine and in implementing hygienic measures in army hospitals to prevent the spread of infection. She clashed with Florence Nightingale when she took up her work in the Crimea.

Barry campaigned against slavery and for the improvement of conditions in lunatic asylums, maintaining they were bad enough to drive a sane person insane. She was outspoken in her criticism of army medical care and was finally posted to the tropics to cause less embarrassment to army personnel.

Her practice of medicine, which emphasized hygiene and the preventive side of health care, exemplifies the special approach of the woman healer. Also of interest was her involvement in politics and her desire that the public be better informed about their bodies in order to make better choices about health care.

When she died in 1865, it was revealed that she was a woman. This caused a sensation, especially in the light of her reputation as a lady-killer. Her medical achievements have not been recognized as a result of the shock and outrage following the discovery of her sex.

As the nineteenth century closed, women doctors, both orthodox and unorthodox, were beginning to reclaim the status and prestige they had had in the past. Women were allowed access to worlds effectively closed to them since the time of the Inquisition.

# 9

# $\mathcal{P}$ersecution Through Committee

WOMEN PRACTITIONERS, FROM REGISTRAR TO CONSULTANT, can be found in any hospital ward or doctors' surgery in Britain today, although female consultants are scarce. And women are members of all the professional bodies, although not welcome in all of their meeting places: "[Women are] Excluded from the cosy male get-togethers where, it is rumoured, all the consultant posts are 'fixed.'"[1]

Although the majority of both conventional and alternative practitioners are white and middle class, theoretically, medical education is open to everyone. But once in practice, women and black men are expected to be better than their white male counterparts, to work harder for the same rewards, to do the dirtier and less glamorous jobs, and to keep their heads down. When a woman is seen to be threatening the male orthodoxy and taking the initiative rather than following established procedures, it can have serious consequences for her professional and personal life. As a consultant wrote about Wendy Savage's behavior in the mid-1980s:

> She should have been a good and agreeable girl and made sure she got on with her colleagues. If she had played her cards right she would have found being a woman was to her advantage and her male colleagues might have been prepared to do her more favours.[2]

That is, if she had been seductive and had used feminine wiles rather than being assertive and using direct action, Wendy Savage might have got what she had wanted without fuss.

Today, women are physicians, just as they have always been, and they are persecuted just as much as they have been in the past. A knowledge of history helps to put current struggles into perspective, so that we remain conscious and aware that the struggles will probably never be over until patriarchy and the domination of white male values comes to an end.

# JILLY ROSSER AND THE INDEPENDENT MIDWIVES

Independent midwives work outside the UK National Health Service (NHS), delivering babies in the mothers' homes. They work in tandem with general practitioners (GPs), if the latter are willing. Midwifery in England has only just survived the onslaught of obstetricians; as Wendy Savage has suggested, "it looks like the midwifery hierarchy is going to finish off what the obstectricians began."[3]

Midwifery has always been seen as female territory, and therefore a threat to male medicine. Male midwifery heralded the beginning of obstetrics and gynecology, and obstetrics is now the most lucrative of all the specialities. In many western countries, only doctors can practice midwifery and lay midwives are illegal. The Peel Report of 1970, which was accepted by the Royal College of Obstetricians, suggested that the UK should aim for 100 percent hospital births. Independent midwives, however, see themselves as professionals in their own right. The majority left the NHS because they did not agree with the way the service managed births within hospital obstetric units. A woman within the NHS, for instance, might see up to fifteen different midwives during her pregnancy. There is no continuity of treatment, and women often feel confused and alienated from health professionals. The midwives themselves feel the lack of continuity and are frustrated by the fragmentary approach within the NHS. An independent midwife takes the initial consultation in the woman's home, which may last up to three hours and include a complete social and medical history. The midwife then supervises the woman throughout her pregnancy, during the birth, and afterward. These services are expensive, but many women feel the financial sacrifice is worthwhile if they can have a peaceful pregnancy and a birth in a nourishing environment.

Because of the threat they are under from outside their profession, many midwives are very protective of their professional status. They do not see why they should be treated differently from doctors undergoing disciplinary procedures. Pending investigation for supposed medical misconduct, midwives are suspended immediately, thus losing their incomes. They are punished before being found guilty. The NHS midwifery supervisors maintain that independent midwives have to work within a code of practice and that often there is misunderstanding between midwife and supervisor. They are more likely to use natural birth methods than state midwives. There is no unanimity about the correct way to manage labor.

Jilly Rosser was struck off the UK Central Council for Nursing, Midwifery and Health Visiting (UKCC) on 10 September 1988, despite her previous good character. She was found guilty on four charges of misconduct. She was punished before she was tried. As an independent midwife, she was prevented from working, and she herself estimated she lost £10,000 in fees for the year it took her case to come before the professional conduct committee.

Rosser was charged with taking a mother and baby to the hospital in her own car, without resuscitation equipment or additional professional help; not waiting for the emergency services when the mother began to hemorrhage; and failing to call the emergency obstetric unit or a registered medical practitioner after her patient's condition had deteriorated. Rosser claimed she tried without success to contact the woman's GP and was concerned that the obstetric flying squad would not arrive in time to save her life. (This was a real possibility owing to the cutbacks in NHS services.) The other charges were failing to make adequate records of observations and the care given and failing to carry out the examinations necessary to determine the cause of the deterioration.

No one was quite sure why the case had been brought before the disciplinary committee. All the witnesses, except one (including the prosecution witnesses) agreed that under similar circumstances they would have made the same decisions.

> If a practitioner is shown previously to be blameless, is moving towards improving his or her practice, has subsequently acted to protect the client, and has demonstrably suffered financially or otherwise as a result of being investigated, should such a practitioner be punished for his or her error of judgement?[4]

Clearly the UKCC felt so. As Luke Zander, an obstetrician and a GP, pointed out in a letter to the *British Medical Journal*:

> Judgement seemed to be based on the extent to which certain procedures had been followed rather than on why and whether the actions taken might have been appropriate or at least justifiable in that particular situation.[5]

And judgment seems to have run contrary to the code of practice for the UKCC, which states:

> The standard of practice in the delivery of midwifery care shall be that which is acceptable in the context of current medical knowledge and clinical developments. In all circumstances, the welfare of the woman and/or her baby must be of primary importance.[6]

Clearly, Rosser was following this code by taking a pregnant woman to the hospital in the quickest way possible so that she might not die from a hemorrhage.

Rosser appealed against the UKCC decision and the judge was unequivocal in support of her actions. He remarked: "We all make mistakes—even lawyers and doctors make mistakes, but we are not struck off for them."[7]

Her supporters hoped the judge would make a judgment defining the concept of misconduct, but the case was stopped before he summed up as the prosecuting barrister conceded the case on the second day of the hearing. The judge was critical of the term misconduct and felt that what was expected of midwives was unrealistic. When discussing how Rosser was accused of not taking adequate notes, he read them and remarked that they were satisfactory, while wryly pointing out the impossibility of taking copious notes when attending to a hemorrhaging woman, phoning the emergency services, and preparing to take her to the hospital. The barrister for the UKCC, in suggesting she could have been taking notes while holding the mother's hand, caused laughter in the court and the judge to observe that "she would have to be a first class juggler." Rosser won her appeal and costs against the UKCC. It was clear that "the UKCC capitulated because it was justifiably in fear of what would come out in the judgement; it was an exercise in damage limitation."[8]

Rosser was not the only independent midwife under investigation in the late 1980s. Caroline Flint was being investigated by the English Board for Nursing and Midwifery and Health Visiting because she wrote an article in the *Nursing Times* about different ways of managing births and mentioned a case of her own, thus breaching confidentiality regulations. Another midwife, Gwen Atkinson, was under a six-month suspension from the South East Thames Regional Health Authority after a difficult birth, while a NHS community midwife was dismissed for failing to report for work at her hospital and for calling a second midwife to back her up. In each of the complaints the outcome for the mother and baby was satisfactory. Caroline Flint says that there have been several other cases in which midwives have been investigated at the local level, "but because of the recent publicity their accusers— often senior midwives—have backed off." She sees the conflicts as part of an attempt by the medical profession and the midwifery hierarchy to control births at home.[9]

Of the seventy registered independent midwives in the UK, most of whom practice in London, seven were subject to disciplinary action in 1988. Beverley Beech of the Association for the Improvement of Midwifery Services (AIMS) believes there is a conspiracy against midwives,[10] and it would appear from the number of cases under investigation that this might well be the case. It seems that midwives who practice outside the NHS are viewed within the midwifery hierarchy as a threat or challenge; they are mavericks who do not fit in the system. Perhaps there is professional jealousy and fear of women having too much autonomy and power in a field where traditional male values hold sway and men make all the decisions.

This struggle will continue as more and more women opt for home births outside the NHS and midwives become increasingly disenchanted with the way that births are managed in hospitals. Midwives working at home are far removed from the control of obstetricians and senior midwives; acting autonomously, they are able to conduct their professional expertise without being supervised by the more conservative elements in midwifery. And such women might be perceived to be dangerous.

## WENDY SAVAGE AND TOWER HAMLETS

In the case of Wendy Savage, a consultant obstetrician and senior lecturer in obstetrics at the London Hospital, two words were constantly applied to both her and her practice: dangerous and threatening.

Savage was suspended from her post as honorary NHS consultant in obstetrics and gynecology at the Tower Hamlets Health Authority on 24 April 1985 on the grounds of alleged incompetence. She had been in practice for twenty-five years. Although the suspension came as a complete surprise to her, there had been repeated problems between her and her professor who worked at the London Hospital.

> This battle was about the way doctors related to and work with each other, and about the fact that I am not a member of the "establishment" and saw no reason to conform to the medical profession's unwritten, but well understood "party line," especially if I thought this was not in the interests of patients.[11]

Savage was given twenty-four hours' notice of the suspension by telephone. Some of her case notes had been taken without her knowledge, an ethically dubious move, and sent to the assessor for infant mortality. She was told that she could not continue with her teaching work at London University, the implication being that if she was incompetent clinically she was not fit to teach medical students.

Suspension of a consultant is usually only considered when emergency measures need to be taken to protect a doctor from harming patients because of mental illness, drugs, or alcohol abuse. To consider suspension of a consultant on the basis of five of her worst cases is as extreme as it is unreasonable. But it started an inquiry that lasted fifteen months, cost an already overstretched Tower Hamlets Health Authority over £250,000, and ended by resolving nothing.

Why was Wendy Savage put through her ordeal both by committee and the media? In her own words: "I and many of my supporters saw my suspension as part of the continuing struggle about who controls childbirth, and it was on this ground that we chose to fight."[12] She continues: "this isn't about competence, it's about attitudes, about a different approach to maternity care."[13]

Many of Savage's attitudes toward obstetrics and gynecology were at variance with the orthodoxy. One was over the issue of abortions. Because of experiences she had had as a medical student of seeing women die as a result of botched abortions, she became a firm supporter of a woman's right to choose. Her experiences in Africa compounded this belief, especially in the light of the hypocritical attitudes of her colleagues. She said: "Why did some of my medical colleagues . . . lie to me about their illegal abortion activities, and appear to forget medical ethics when money was involved?"[14]

An abortion center was set up using nonmedical counselors, and the clinic provided an out-patient abortion facility for women who were healthy and less than thirteen weeks pregnant. Some of her colleagues were very unhappy about this and claimed it made Tower Hamlets the abortion capital of London. It was believed that some of their animosity toward her stemmed from this.[15]

Choice in childbirth was another contentious issue. Savage and her team encouraged GPs to be involved and for midwives to do home delivery services with hospital backup. They tried to get a GP unit for deliveries in the London Hospital, but this was blocked by other consultants.

What our colleagues appeared to dislike most is that we offered the GPs choice. They felt that the consultant should take the decision about the woman's delivery. Fundamentally, the issue was power . . .[16]

Her views on pregnancy also caused concern, if not panic, among her fellow consultants:

Pregnancy is not an illness. I belong to the school of thought which believes that every pregnancy is normal unless there are indications that something is wrong . . . if you look at each woman as an individual, and plan her care with her, you will get the best result.[17]

The issue of birth and power is one which arouses strong emotions, because birth is a profoundly moving experience. . . . Birth arouses primitive and elemental feelings within us. . . . It reminds us of death as well as life.[18]

That is, it reminds the physician that in some situations, he or she is powerless. One baby in every hundred dies in the uterus or in the first week of life, and obstetricians will see on average five to ten women every year who leave the hospital without a live baby. A different course of action might have saved a quarter or a half of those babies, and guilt feelings and other unpleasant emotions can be overwhelming.

Savage summed up her beliefs as follows:

involving the woman in the decisions about her care, means the obstetrician must relinquish some power. Accepting that the woman should have some control over her own fertility . . . seems to be deeply threatening to some obstetricians of both sexes.[19]

She also points out that the majority of consultants are men, whereas all the consumers are women and that: "The role of the doctor is that of counsellor rather than that of an authoritarian, trained professional, and this is very hard for some doctors to accept—especially the majority of male obstetricians."[20]

The extreme action of having Wendy Savage suspended, with the possibility of losing not only her job but the right to practice her profession, can only be described as outrageous. As one journalist remarked:

> Some doctors who complain vociferously about trial by the media are themselves active proponents of that traditional medical pastime, trial by gossip. . . . The gossip . . . included allegations about Mrs Savage's sexual inclinations and marital history.[21]

The difference in what women want from obstetrics and what the medical profession feels inclined to give them can be seen in the different responses given by the CTPs and Fellows of the Royal College of Obstetricians and Gynaecologists. The doctors, health workers, and women's health groups rallied round Savage from the outset and set in motion a support campaign. They began fund-raising to pay the costs of her court case. She received over twenty letters of support from GPs and midwives in the first four days after her suspension, yet only a handful of hospital doctors and medical college staff wrote to her. Medical students were also very supportive and several joined the support group and organized private lectures before their finals. Over eighty GPs in Tower Hamlets signed the petition, which explained why there was no problem about her returning to the area to work after she had been cleared. The support at the grass-roots level was enormous.

The legal battle commenced in February 1986, and the court case lasted over three weeks. Like the battle medical women faced a century previously, public pressure was important. Savage's lawyer, Brian Raymond, stated: "Your power in the court is directly proportional to your power outside the court." [22]

The five incidents were selected from over eight hundred cases of women who had had babies under the care of Savage in the period from 1983 to 1984. Four of the deliveries were very unusual.

In the first case the woman concerned was allowed to continue for too long in the second stage of labor, particularly as it was a breech birth. The treatment was idiosyncratic, but the assessment was deemed to be correct. In the second case the baby failed to thrive. The third case involved a Bangladeshi woman who had had a cesarean with her first delivery and for her second wanted a normal delivery for a variety of social, religious, and cultural reasons. She was allowed to be in labor until such time as it became clear that a vaginal birth was not possible and a cesarean was then performed. The mother and baby were well, but ten days after the birth the baby died from a blood disorder, which, it was maintained, was caused by pressure it had received during labor. Although there was no evidence to suppose that the management of the birth caused the baby's death, it was considered an unwise choice of treatment. The fourth case involved a mother of twins who developed serious anemia, which was not treated in time, resulting in a severe eclampsia. The mother wanted to try for a normal delivery, and Savage agreed, but later elected for a cesarean. The criticism here was that she should not have done so. Both mother and twins are fine. The final case also necessitated a cesarean, which Savage was reluctant to order early on in the labor. When the time came for the operation, she did not personally supervise the house doctor who performed it.

None of the charges were severe; as one of her witnesses remarked:

> In a busy hospital misjudgements, failures in communication and frank mistakes are bound to occur to the best of doctors. It is usual to show understanding and sympathy when such events occur to a colleague, yet I find no trace of such support. . . . In no case is Dr. Savage given the benefit of the doubt.[23]

In summing up, the prosecution had to resort to character assassination. It was claimed the junior staff were terrified of Savage, that she was a crusader, had "perhaps a sharp temper," and had a grave defect of character, "which is an inability to recognise fault in one's self."[24]

The conclusion of the medical panel was that Savage revealed a consistent aberration of judgment and that in only one case did she come close to the bounds of acceptable practice. An editorial in the

*British Medical Journal* concluded: "Mrs Savage's strongly held and voiced opinions on women's rights to a say in their method of delivery and their rights to abortion made her a public and at times controversial figure."[25] But it should be borne in mind that: "The medical profession still behaves on occasions like an Edwardian gentleman's club, concerned to close ranks against anyone with nonconformist tendencies and taking on faith the integrity of 'clubbable' individuals."[26]

Many professionals expressed shame at the response of the medical profession and at the Royal College for not speaking up in her defense. Dr. Anthony Clare, professor of psychological medicine at St. Bartholomew's Hospital, wrote:

> Throughout all this the London Hospital Medical College stood aloof, although one of its professors was publicly accusing one of its senior lecturers of incompetence. A better example of the current spinelessness of much of academic medicine would be hard to find . . . . [If] there is a moral, and I suspect there are a few, it is that if doctors yield their right to regulate themselves up to administrators, managers and lawyers, then such claim as they have to be a profession disappears. And they should not be surprised if the dignity, the standing and the respect that a profession commands disappears with it.[27]

An editorial in the *Lancet* follows in a similar vein:

> With a few honourable exceptions, doctors have been silent; and one gloomy interpretation is that, in a profession built on patronage, individuals are hesitant to "put their head over the parapet." The Royal College of Obstetricians and Gynaecologists is deeply involved. Yet we have heard almost nothing from that quarter. Its officials seem to have been more concerned with maintaining a semblance of decorum than with intervening in a matter of justice and principle.[28]

It might be argued that the case brought the debate about childbirth and family planning services into the open and showed the public how far the majority of obstetricians and gynecologists are from their way of thinking.

Savage was reinstated in her position as honorary NHS consultant at Tower Hamlets and today continues her pioneering work.

## DR. MARIETTA HIGGS AND THE CLEVELAND CASE

In 1987 a crisis erupted in the northern county of Cleveland (U.K.) that undermined some basic assumptions held by society regarding family life. Between spring and early summer of that year, 121 children in the Cleveland area, with an average age of seven, were diagnosed as having been sexually abused. They were diagnosed by two pediatricians, Dr. Marietta Higgs and Dr. Geoffrey Wyatt. After many months of legal wrangling, it was decided that twenty-six of these children had been incorrectly diagnosed.

The alarm expressed by the public and voiced through the tabloid press was that the two women at the center of the case, Marietta Higgs and Sue Richardson, the senior social worker, were allowed to continue working with sexual abuse cases. The issue of protecting the rights of children and babies was lost in a hysterical outcry against these two women professionals. The affair culminated in an inquiry chaired by a woman judge, Lord Justice Butler-Sloss, which cost around £2 million.[29]

The degree of public outcry had more to do with the nature of the crime, that is, sex, than with the crime itself. In our society, sex remains a taboo subject, in spite of the so-called sexual revolution. Sex between adults and children, especially between fathers and their children, is a: "crime committed by men, notably fathers, against women and children."[30] The recognition of sexual abuse challenges men and is a political threat because men are the abusers and men by and large have the job of investigating and punishing those responsible. The police reacted to the Higgs case with "masculine panic, then tantrums and a reliance on 'masculine intuition,' all of which became palpable in the police evidence to the inquiry."[31]

The case is complex. It involves the medical profession, represented by the two pediatricians, protecting children, and, it is claimed, over-reacting to the probable existence of sexual abuse, along with the social services who also defended the children, notably Sue Richardson and her boss, Mike Bishop, the director. Then there are the police doctors, Irvine and Roberts, who opposed the diagnoses, the local Labour MP, Stuart Bell, and the Reverend Michael Wright, who defended the fathers.

Until recently, sexual abuse of children was thought to exist only in situations of poverty and ignorance. It has now become apparent, however, that it occurs in all types of families, crossing class, race, religious, and ethnic lines. Fathers, step-fathers, uncles, and family friends are often the perpetrators, and children of both sexes, from babies of six months and younger to seventeen-year-olds are the victims. As Beatrix Campbell maintains: "Doing something about sexual abuse presents a poignant challenge to society, politically and professionally."[32]

Higgs was castigated by the press for being cold, contained, disciplined, rational—all the qualities with which men are identified. The police, however, were perceived to have behaved irrationally, to have acted on hunches, and to have had gut feelings. As one police inspector remarked: "Sexual abuse is like a corpse on a slab, saying nothing. You've got nothing to go on. It's a police officer's nightmare. You just want it to go away."[33]

Once the crisis was underway and the children's ward of Middlesborough General Hospital began to fill up with children suspected of having been abused; the trouble began. Nurses, already overstretched, could not cope with these children and their outraged parents arrived on the wards picking fights, crying, arguing, and sometimes staying in the adjoining parents' room. Higgs was unmoved by the nurses' appeals to slow down the referrals. The police refused to take on cases diagnosed by her unless substantiated by other physicians. They maintained there was a conspiracy going on between Higgs and Richardson.

Wright, who started and coordinated the Fathers' Support Group, believed a feminist mafia was operating in Cleveland and that a lot of the women felt their families would be better off without fathers. (This in fact would surely be the opinion of any mother who felt the father of her children was sexually abusing them.)

Higgs enraged the police and those who disagreed with her because: "They could not *force* her to change her mind."[34] She was convinced she was right and that, like the children who had been abused, no one believed what she was saying. But her strength of character and belief in her diagnosis made her an unshakable force. And her courage to go against her colleagues who wanted her to take a more reasonable approach was remarkable. One colleague agreed with her diagnoses but said many doctors would hesitate to call in the social services knowing the work that was involved once a case was diagnosed. Higgs was told to wait until there were better facilities for looking after the children. But she would not.

Her colleagues supported her, but as one remarked: "She tried to do the right thing the wrong way."[35] And it is clear she lacked the support of the staff with whom she worked; no support committee was formed, unlike that for Wendy Savage. Her personality may have had something to do with the lack of support, but the issue of sexual abuse also determined how she was treated. Savage engendered the patriarchal wrath of gynecologists, but Higgs took on the very foundation of patriarchal society: the family. As Dr. Jane Wynne, a pediatrician from Leeds, remarked: "If you accept that child sexual abuse happens then you accept that there must be a lot of adults abusing, and it starts to say something about our society: who we are, the way we live, and the way we treat each other."[36]

It is hardly surprising, therefore, that politicians and patriarchal forces such as the church rebelled. The implications of the case were immense. Wyatt remarked to the inquiry that unless the status of women and children in our society changed, the situation would never improve.

Sadly, the inquiry did not look at causes, but instead concentrated on symptoms and children's bodies. It was impossible during the inquiry to suggest that an epidemic of sexual abuse meant there had to be an epidemic of abusers.

In this case, a woman in a position of power and authority defended the defenseless against men, the rapists. But in a skillful about-face, the accuser became the accused, and all the hatred, bigotry and abuse that patriarchy has at its disposal were directed at the woman.

> The open hostilities in Cleveland between social services and the
> police became a war of the sexes. . . . What was worrying was the
> obvious lack of objectivity on the part of Mrs Richardson. . . . She
> openly supported Dr Higgs 100 per cent.[37]

These remarks were made by Police Inspector Makepeace who was at
a meeting on May 28 during which Dr. Alistair Irvine, the police
surgeon, shouted at Higgs in an effort to break her in time-honored
police fashion. Higgs, however, remained calm, answered his questions politely, and enraged the good doctor to such an extent that he
stormed out of the meeting. Makepeace commented that "I would not
like to give the impression that Dr. Irvine lost all sense of control."[38]
Irvine had told Higgs that she was incompetent, disparaged her diagnosis, and threatened writs. The following day the police informed
social services that there would be no more meetings between them.
In effect, they broke off all contact and precipitated the crisis.

The police critique of both Richardson and Higgs reveals the key
issues:

> stubborn, obsessed, besotted, neurotic, knowing witches versus
> the common-sensical bobby. . . . All these terms, of course,
> described the opposite: the women were sombre, rational, calm.
> And what was perhaps unforgivable, they knew more than their
> police protagonists. The women just sat there while bombastic
> men threw tantrums and threatened.[39]

The interrogation of the social workers at the inquiry also highlighted
the situation. Some were even questioned about their personal lives,
their families, to which political party they belonged, and one was
asked if she was married, which had never happened before in any
court case. Thus the women found themselves to be women first and
professionals a poor second, a vivid reminder of the witch trials and
the accusations against women throughout the centuries.

The inquiry acknowledged the dedication and commitment shown by Higgs and Richardson. Higgs was criticized for relying solely on physical findings to make her diagnosis and for not taking a leadership role. It was agreed she had difficult working relationships with her staff, but no one person was to blame for this. Irvine, the police surgeon, was criticized for his poor relations with the social workers and for the lack of communication. This caused all parties to lose sight of the abused children who should have been at the center of the dispute.

Higgs and Wyatt were suspended from their work at Middlesborough General Hospital. Wyatt eventually returned to work at the hospital, but Higgs was put through a further ordeal of disciplinary action by the Northern Region Health Authority, which tried to stop her from ever again working with sex abuse cases, to ban her from working in Cleveland, to end her secondment in Newcastle, and to give her a serious reprimand. The authority refused to hold an inquiry into her alleged professional misconduct, and Higgs was forced to take the case to the High Court. But she failed to stop the disciplinary action.

> Whatever our opinions, all of us must have sympathised with Dr Higgs as she become the target of intrusive and hostile reporting, with stringers in Australia detailed to dig for skeletons in her family cupboard.
>
> Curiously, Dr Wyatt was handled less roughly. Was this because he is less tantalising to journalists than an apparently self-possessed woman whom they were unable to intimidate? Or was it because he is not a woman? . . . [T]hey love a villain and powerful women are more likely to be cast in this role than equally powerful men.[40]

# 10

# *W*omen Shamans and Conjurers

LOOKING AT THE PRACTICE OF CONTEMPORARY WOMEN shamans and conjurers points to a living tradition, unbroken for thousands of years, with knowledge passed down from mother to daughter by word of mouth through the telling of myths and fables. Their medicine is generally practiced in secret as these women have been persecuted for their skills. They are older women who enjoy a high status in their communities and are treated as honorary men. For this reason they are both respected and feared.

Seeing a traditional healer at work brings us full circle in the history of women in medicine. Reconnecting with these healing foremothers is a liberating and empowering experience for women, as both patients and practitioners.

Crones, that is, women past the age of childbearing and childrearing, have the time and energy to devote to their work, which is not possible for a mother with small children. They also no longer menstruate, and therefore cannot be seen to be a polluting force.[1]

A crone, as defined in Vicki Noble's *Motherpeace,* is: "the old wise woman who watches over our dreams and visions. . . . The Crone is the Hag who knows how to call down the power of the moon, to converse with spirits and work magical spells."[2]

Eric Neumann, in his opus *The Great Mother,* discusses the female shaman.[3] Shamans often have many things in common. A variety of debilitating factors such as repeated childbearing, sickness, menstruation, and hunger develops the character of the shaman. Many first realize their gifts after a severe illness, a period of madness, or great privation. Such tests develop the character, stamina, and willpower. A shaman needs to have discipline, self-control, and fierce determination to overcome whatever obstacles are put in her way. This prepares the initiate for the severe trials of strength she will encounter in magical rites and rituals. Initiation may be associated with sickness and deprivation, or it may involve the taking of hallucinogenic drugs, such as opium or certain herbs or other mind-altering substances. Fasting is also used to change consciousness. Drumming, dancing, and chanting are important tools in any healing ritual, and special songs and chants are handed down from mother to daughter to be used during these ceremonies. The use of hallucinogenic substances have traditionally formed part of a wise woman's repertoire and are the natural province of woman. Neumann remarks:

> All these aids merely set in motion a natural potency of the
> female psyche, through which from time immemorial woman,
> in her character of shaman, sibyl, priestess, and wise woman, has
> influenced mankind.[4]

Woman was the original seer, lady of the waters of the night, watcher of the seasons, listener to the moon and stars. She is overpowered by the spirit that erupts and speaks through her. She becomes the center of magical song and poetry. It is as if "every cell can be alive and vibrating as if one were electrical or indescribably blissful."[5]

Four components are usually to be found in the actual treatment process.[6] First, there has to be a special place for healing to take place. In ancient times, this was the temple, whether that of Isis, Hecate at the crossroads, or Diana in the hills. A place was set aside and an atmosphere created that was conducive to healing. The atmosphere is most important. The place can be very basic, but the healer has to build up a healing atmosphere that provides an attractive force and at the same time releases and reassures the patient.

Second, a rationale or myth has to explain the suffering of the patient and allow for the possibility of cure. Third, rituals or practices have to overcome suffering by relieving distress and increasing the feeling of well-being. Finally, a relationship of trust must exist between the healer and her client; the client must have confidence that a cure is possible and have faith in a positive outcome.

# THE NATIVE AMERICAN HEALING TRADITION

*And when we hear in the Navajo chant of the mountain that a*
*grown man sits and smokes with bears and follows directions*
*given to him by squirrels, we are surprised. We had thought only*
*little girls spoke with animals.[7]*

Native North Americans are a good example of a people with a culture which has to a large extent withstood the onslaught of Western cultural imperialism. The culture has been able to retain its integrity and a powerful sense of its identity. The history of the Native American nation stretches back as far as Western prehistory, but unlike ancient Greece, Egypt, or Rome, it has managed to withstand and resist a takeover of its culture by the invading and dominating whites, although the sacrifice has at times been enormous.

When whites invaded Native American lands, they found a system of medicine well in advance of their own.

> The average Indian on-the-plains or in-the-woods knew more
> about anatomy and the treatment of trauma and illness than the
> average European, and in some respects, more than European
> physicians. . . . Native American understanding and treatment of
> wounds was far superior to that of whites . . . countless observers
> . . . remarked on the fact that few cripples or amputees were seen
> among the natives.[8]

Indigenous Americans are credited with the invention of the syringe (using an animal bladder bulb and a hollow bone as quill or applicator) and for recognizing the need for draining deep wounds. They are also credited for having paved the way for the discovery of insulin and the birth control pill.[9] Central to their practice of medicine is a deep abiding respect for nature and the earth; a recognition of the importance of community and relationships, together with reverence and attention to the spiritual life. Their system balances the spiritual with the physical, in the form of both attention to the gods and sensible, hygienic practices.

Native Americans' relationship with the earth speaks of this deep spiritual connection, to this our first mother. The earth is like the body of the mother. When encouraged to practice agriculture by the whites, some Native Americans responded with horror; this would be defiling the very body of this most precious woman: mother, wife, sister.

> You ask me to plough the ground! Shall I take a knife and tear my mother's bosom? Then when I die she will not take me to her bosom to rest.
>
> You ask me to dig for stone! Shall I dig under her skin for her bones? Then when I die I cannot enter her body to be born again.[10]

A Pawnee priest describes it thus:

> H'Uraru, the Earth, is very near to man; we speak of her as Atira, Mother, because she brings forth. From the Earth we get our food; we lie down on her; we live and walk on her; we could not exist without her, as we could not breathe without Hoturu, the Winds, or grow without Shakuru, the Sun.[11]

There is a ritual of the Pawnee people called Hako. It is a prayer for life and children, for health and prosperity. It is directed to the universal powers, to father heaven and mother earth. Birds are the intermediaries that fly between these two places. The eagle is the highest of the bird messengers. The ear of corn represents the daughter of heaven and earth, Mother Corn. H'Uraru represents the sacred power that brings forth life and sustains it. The kernel is planted in the earth and brings forth in the same way that a mother does. The priest says: "We give the cry of reverence to Mother Corn, she who brings the promise of children, of strength, of life, of plenty, and of peace."[12]

## Pasowee

The myth of Pasowee, the Buffalo Woman, comes from the Kiowa people, who were believed to have lived in the Wyoming area before they settled in Kansas and Oklahoma. It is said that this myth is related to one of the sacred societies of the Kiowa, the Buffalo Women. This sacred society of women is especially associated with ritual dance and healing.

Pasowee was stolen from her family in the middle of the night and spent many years living with the strangers. One day, driven by despair at being separated from her loved ones, she ran off into the woods and escaped. She ran and ran, and exhausted toward the end of the day, she came upon the hide of a long-dead buffalo. Creeping under its skin, she lay down to sleep and dreamed the whole night. The buffalo came to her and told of his magic; of cures that could be found within his body and how to use them to heal the sick. The buffalo whispered the wisdom of the ages to Pasowee.

The next morning, Pasowee awoke and saw two wolves kill a buffalo, just as her dream had predicted. When they had eaten their fill, Pasowee took some of the meat and dried it. When it was dry, she continued on her journey to find her people. When finally she arrived at her family's camp, she showed them a piece of buffalo hide that she had brought with her. Drying it over hot stones, she stitched it together to make a deep pouch. In that pouch she put the medicine that had been made known to her in her sleep. The buffalo medicine brought joy and good health to her people.[13]

## Annie Kahn

Annie Kahn is a Navajo healer. She was given her name by whites, who could not or would not use her Native American name. She is also called the "Flower that speaks the pollen way." Annie Kahn was initiated in the medicine traditions while still in her mother's womb. A ceremony known as the Blessingway was held with a medicine man praying over her pregnant mother. While still a developing fetus, her parents taught her the secrets of medicine, which she describes: "They talked medicine. . . . They went out there to touch and talk and pace and shake it in their ear. They prepared."[14]

Her parents taught her about the harmony that exists in nature as a way of preparing her for her birth. They told her stories of plants, of spirits, and of her ancestors and taught her about the four souls each person has and the mysteries of the Navajo culture. After she was born and while growing up, both her parents and her grandparents taught her. They used the cycle of nature to illustrate their teachings and encouraged her to use her five senses to connect with the things she saw, felt, heard, touched, and tasted. As a child she memorized this learning, as memory is a vital part of the training. Knowledge is learned from the outside, but when working with it, it has to come from the inside. For example, she was given a flower to taste so that she might forever have a connection with that flower. Concentration is also vital for a shaman, the ability to focus without distraction on a task. Concentration is a precursor to meditation or deep thought.

Talking of her ideas about illness, Kahn says:

> You are sick when you develop the habit of excluding. Therefore, you are off balance. You're out of harmony. Everything that interferes with living makes illness. The mind and the body interaction during physical illness causes a friction and lack of cooperation. The mind is to tell the body what to do. But if the mind is either too fast or too slow, the body may describe and reveal what the mind is doing. . . . Not accepting causes illness. Causes delay. Therefore there is friction causing greater illness. To heal, one must be in balance. Must understand. Must accept. This very act causes healing.[15]

Kahn discusses the agents that bring about healing: consciousness-raising, organization and order, obedience and faith, power and spirituality, preparation for the ceremony, and the healing ceremony itself. Her treatment is truly holistic. The healer first works to increase the

awareness of the sick person. Kahn describes how she raises consciousness by wearing a beautiful necklace. Beauty lifts the spirit and shows
peace and quiet. As the patient sees this beauty outside herself, she is
reminded of her inner beauty and is encouraged to search it out. The
attitude of the patient is paramount in the healing process. Likewise,
obedience and discipline are prerequisites for the cure. Obedience is

> submission to the laws of order, while discipline is the self-
> control and efficiency that enforces obedience. There is always a
> maturity of attitude involved and it is continuous. Like a diet. It
> is personal, gentle, peaceful.[16]

The role of faith is to establish sincerity and dedication. Trust and
obedience are developed to engender respect for the cycles of time and
the rhythms of life.

Kahn prepares for a healing ceremony in the following way. She
gets up at five in the morning to tell the earth and the sky about the
person who is coming. As a conductor of healing energy, but not its
originator, she opens herself up to the forces in her environment, the
powers of mother earth and father sky. She needs the healing energy
from the earth and from the sky. She speaks to her ancestors, tapping
into their knowledge. She washes her hair to ensure that her head is
cool and calm for the healing ceremony. She makes sure she is free
from her menstrual period, as the blood is seen to be polluting. She
collects the plants she needs and decides how much consciousness-
raising she needs to do. Thus prepared, she meets her patient. The
questions she asks her clients indicate how far-reaching her diagnosis
and treatment will be. She asks her clients why they are sick, a very
important question. (As a healer myself, I have discovered that most
people know why they are ill; they just need to be given the opportunity to think about it.) Kahn asks what kind of food her clients eat,
what they do, what they hide from themselves, and what they do not
tell their regular doctors. She listens to the replies and notes what the
clients leave unsaid—the spaces between the words. And from all of
this she arrives at her diagnosis. Each prescription in the Blessingway
is personal. A medicine woman who specializes in herbal remedies

might be hired to make up a special herbal mixture. The patient is given a plant to take home with him or her, to hold, to see, to talk, to taste. This allows the patient to become acquainted with herbs.

The recovery comes from inside. Kahn says that: "Spirituality is healing. Spirituality is power. No medicine woman will say that she has power because the power belongs to the great spirit. It is not hers.[17]. . . Buffalo Woman assists in the healing ritual. Buffalo has a sacred name and White Buffalo is healing power. . . . What makes a medicine woman a medicine woman? The White Buffalo."[18]

Thus the Navajo medicine woman, like the ancient Egyptians and Greeks, will call on the gods or the spirits to help her heal.

## SERBIAN CONJURERS

Serbian women conjurers form part of an ancient healing tradition that originates in central Serbia. It is believed their healing practices go back to very ancient times,[19] that is, they predate Christianity and also the patriarchal Roman gods. Their healing rituals are full of the imagery of the mother, perhaps referring back to the Great Mother, and the chants and songs also echo this theme. The teaching of this tradition is matrilineal, going from mother to daughter, grandmother to grandchild. In this tradition only postmenopausal women may use the learned material. Women and girls of any age may study the healing methods, but the practice is reserved exclusively for women who have finished menstruating.

These women live in an extremely patriarchal society. The men control the means of production and both secular and ritual life. They perform the rituals for daily, seasonal, and annual events. But the women conjurers perform rituals for individuals. Until they can no longer reproduce, the women's lives are tightly controlled by the men. Once postmenopausal, women are accorded the status of honorary men. They can go out at night, swear, drink, behave outrageously—and they can conjure.

The men see the women as a polluting force. Their menstrual blood is believed to have malevolent powers that corrupt, taint, and harm objects and people who come into contact with it. At puberty, with their first period, the girls of the village are taught about the menstrual taboos and the need to isolate themselves to avoid contaminating their environment. Menstrual blood is believed to defile crops, harm livestock, and sap the power of men. Before she can heal, a woman needs to be ritually clean, that is, her menstruation has to have ceased, and then she is no longer a wild, untameable force. Once a crone, she has access to places previously off-limits. She is given power and status in the community, above and beyond that of mother and the breeder of future generations. Nevertheless, as a woman, she still represents the dark chthonic forces. It is she who talks with the dead and is concerned with funerary ritual, she who can tame malevolent spirits and venture into the future, battling ill winds and dark, mysterious forces. She is both the good mother and the terrible destroyer.

Payment for her services is in goods and services, never in cash. Everyone knows who the conjurers are, but no one alludes to them. Their work is carried out in secret, and they are treated with respect and circumspection. Patients do not discuss their treatment as they fear the magic may go wrong if they talk. There is a great fear that the evil eye might fall on their treatment and affect the magic. Men and women consult the conjurers in equal numbers, but conjurers' patients are kept very secret.

## Desanka

Desanka is a Serbian conjurer. To heal a case of erysipelas, she dispels the color red, which represents the inflammation of the skin, by recollecting and inventing metaphors of the red animal mother who provides nourishment for her red young in the unknown world of the *otud* (from out there) where redness belongs. In the real world, such redness is undesirable. Desanka becomes a non-red mother who nurses the red (ill) patient with a non-red charm. When the redness goes, the illness is cured.

One of Desanka's favorite metaphors is that of the red mother hen.

> *From out there comes a red hen*
> *She leads nine red chicks*
> *She fell upon a red dung heap.*[20]

From here she goes on to create another red mother image: a red cow who gives birth to a red calf, a red sow with piglets, a red ewe with a red lamb. The metaphor is of a mother suckling her young, giving healing, nurturing, and life-essence to her young. A home is created in otud for the inappropriate redness, which is the illness; the redness is then dispatched to its home.

Desanka sings a purification refrain when she calls upon the forces of chaos to listen to her and to leave the patient light as a feather (she holds up a feather), as pure as silver (she holds up a silver coin), and as gentle as mother's milk (she cups her hands over her breasts). At the same time, she applies simple herbal remedies to the client that alleviate the physical symptoms of the disease, washing the inflamed skin with home-brewed plum brandy, covering the wound with an ointment based on camphor, and finally bandaging the area with sterile bandages. After a prescribed time, the disease begins to subside.

Conjuring is always done after midday, as the sinking sun carries with it disease and disorder. Although the charms vary considerably in content, an invariable rule specifies that all rituals must be repeated on three successive days. Power is seen to reside in the number three, perhaps reflecting back to the triple mother: maiden, mother, and crone. Thrice three has an even greater significance. Nine-day charms or rituals are extremely powerful. On a more prosaic level, the three days allotted to the charm allow time for the conjurer and the client to bond, which facilitates the healing process.

The nurturing mother image of these conjurers brings us back to the ancient matriarchal past. It also firmly roots women's healing tradition in everyday life. The conjurer does her own work in her own home, all the while carrying on her function as the matriarch of home and community. She is in no way associated with the slick professionalism of male-dominated medicine, rather she is linked to the more homely cures of a local wise woman. People come from far afield to consult her, preferring "her calming voice, the confidence she engenders, and her gentle touch," which are seen to be more attractive than waiting on a bench at the clinic in town.[21]

# $\mathscr{C}$onclusion

THIS BOOK HAS MOVED THROUGH TIME from the very distant prepatriarchal past to the present day. From a world where woman as healer was the norm to a time where women have to fight even to ensure that gentle, holistic methods of treatment have a voice alongside aggressive mechanistic medical techniques.

Increasing numbers of people are dissatisfied with orthodox medicine. People working within this field need to rethink their priorities. The shift in emphasis from art to science during the Renaissance dealt a blow to the tradition of women as healers from which we have yet to recover. In both orthodox and alternative medicine, patriarchal values hold sway. Women are tolerated as long as they do not presume to do anything which might alter the status quo.

The penalties for challenging the medical orthodoxy are severe, as Wendy Savage, Marietta Higgs, and countless other women in medicine will testify. Their crimes, like those of Jacoba Felice in the fourteenth century or Agnodice in ancient Greece, were not of incompetence, abuse, or of being a danger to their patients. They were skilled and innovative practitioners who put the care of their patients first. Their "crime" was that they were women. As healers they should have been lauded rather than disciplined, but they were deemed a threat to the male monopoly within medicine and, as such, a challenge to the stability of patriarchal structures. The full weight of these powerful institutions was pitted against them to ensure their silence.

Hundreds of years have passed since the burning times, the holocaust that killed millions of our women. Progress seems to have been made; women are no longer burned alive or tortured, but the scars remain. I defy any woman to read about the atrocities of the inquisitors and not feel the pain of recognition, the weight of sorrow those women carried, whose burden has been passed to modern women. I defy any woman not to rage at the injustice, the bigotry, and mindless cruelty that is her heritage. Women must be determined to overcome this.

What is the legacy of the holocaust for women healers? I believe that all European women carry a racial memory of those times deep within their psyches. European women have an inordinate and disproportionate fear of public humiliation, which comes from the memory of public strippings, of rapes, torture, and death by burning or drowning. Women have learned the price to be paid if they step too far out of line, if they challenge too openly or get too demanding. Women understand that if they stand up to the establishment, whether church, state, the law, or medicine, they risk their sanity, if not their lives. Prisons, mental institutions, poverty, and tranquilizers are the modern weapons used to curb women's free spirit. The goalposts may have shifted slightly, but the message remains the same: If you make too many waves, you will be at the mercy of those who may at first ridicule you, later pressure you, and ultimately use the law and/or pharmaceuticals to beat you into submission.

Women healers know this. As long as they work within patriarchal structures, whether conventional or alternative, and accept conditions as they are, they are tolerated. But if they push too far, make demands for real change, they see the barriers go up. They become marginalized, silenced by ridicule or contempt; they are starved of cash and resources; they are threatened. All women know this. As physicians and healers they have to juggle in their consciences their desire to do good work with the reality of the marketplace. They have to learn to negotiate the medical minefield. Women healers are learning how to keep their integrity as feminists, and how to do the best for themselves and their clients: how to nurture and be nurtured; how to break down the artificial barriers that exist between healer and patient; how to maintain those barriers that are necessary for their own self-protection; and how to balance material gain with intellectual and emotional output. With the gynocide of the burning times as their legacy, women healers are aware of the need for caution and circumspection, for they understand that misogyny and homophobia are still prevalent. They need to be silent, hidden, and careful—and at the same time outspoken, fearless and inspired. There is much work to be done in researching history and seeking the truth; many wounds need to heal. The process will be long and painful. Women's work as healers can be seen as revolutionary acts. Women healers are here in spite of those who would forbid them, as women fulfilling their instinct to cherish and preserve life.

Women healers have survived and their numbers are growing. In all branches of healing, women are developing their skills and translating their male-identified training in terms of women's experience. Much blood has been shed and yet women are still determined to transcend the sterile plains of intellectualism and weld the art of healing with the science of medicine.

# $\mathscr{N}$otes

## Healing in Antiquity

1 Kate Campbell Hurd-Mead, *A History of Women in Medicine*, 160.

2 Cyril P. Bryan, trans., *The Papyrus Ebers*, 42–43.

3 Dan McKenzie, *The Infancy of Medicine*, 25.

4 See, for instance, F. L. Griffith, *The Petrie Papyri*, 5–ll.

5 Chauncey D. Leake, *The Old Egyptian Medical Papyri*, 8.

6 See Hurd-Mead, *History of Women*, photo facing p. 20.

7 See H. J. Mozans, *Women in Science*, 267.

8 See Hurd-Mead, *History of Women*, 37.

9 Merlin Stone, *Ancient Mirrors of Womanhood*, 203.

10 Hurd-Mead, *History of Women*, 45.

11 Ibid, 40.

12 Mozans, *Women in Science*, 270.

13 Ibid, 271–72.

14 Hurd-Mead, *History of Women*, 54.

15 Ibid, 56.

16 Ibid, 60.

17 Mozans, *Women in Science*, 274.

18 Hurd-Mead, *History of Women*, 79.

19 Mozans, *Women in Science*, 273.

## Medicine in the Dark Ages

1 See chapter 3 in Barbara Walker, *The Woman's Encyclopaedia of Myths and Secrets*.

2 Bryan, trans., *The Papyrus Ebers*, 8.

3 For further information about the gnostic gospels, see Elaine Pagels, *The Gnostic Gospels*.

4 Walker, *Woman's Encyclopaedia*, 208.

5 Ibid, 209.

6 From Martial Book I, F. W. Nicholson, trans. Quoted in Hurd-Mead, *History of Women*.

7 Walker, *Woman's Encyclopaedia*, 211.

8 Muriel Joy Hughes, *Women Healers in Medieval Life and Literature*, 7.

9 See Marion Bradley, *The Mists of Avalon*.

10 See, for instance, Hughes, *Women Healers*.

11 See Eleanour Sinclair Rhode, *The Old English Herbals*.

12 Ibid, 15.

13 Ibid, 18.

## Trotula of Salerno

1 Margaret Alic, *Hypatia's Heritage*, 51.

2 John F. Benton, "Trotula," *Bulletin of the History of Medicine* 59, (1985): 50.

3 Ibid, 50. The story comes from Albertus Magnus, a philosopher and alchemist (1193–1280) who wrote *De Secretis Mulierum*. See also Lynn Thorndike, *A History of Magic and Experimental Science*, vol. 2, 739–45.

4 Alic, *Hypatia's Heritage*, 55.

5 See Edward F. Tuttle, "The Trotula and Old Dame Trot: A Note on the Lady of Salerno," *Bulletin of the History of Medicine* 50 (1976): 62–63.

6 Quoted in Kate Campbell Hurd-Mead, "Trotula," *Isis* 14 (1930): 349.

7 Ibid, 353–54.

8 See Tuttle, "Trotula and Old Dame Trot," 69.

9 From *Placides et Timeo ou Li Secres as Philosophes* (Geneva Librairie Droz: Textes Litteraires Francais, 1980) 133–34, quoted in Benton, "Trotula," 51.

10 Benton, "Trotula," 48–49.

11 See Charles and Dorothea Singer, "Essays in the History of Medicine Presented to Karl Sudhoff," an article on the origin of the medical school of Salerno (Oxford: Oxford University Press, 1924) 129.

12 Hurd-Mead, "Trotula," 364.

13 Elizabeth Mason-Hohl, trans., *The Diseases of Women by Trotula of Salerno: A Translation of Passionibus Mulierum Curandorum*.

14 For an explanation of the four humors and their actions on the body, see Elisabeth Brooke, *A Woman's Book of Herbs*, 3–6.

15 Taken from Salvatore De Renzi, *Collectio Salernitana*, vol. 5, 1852–59, 300–304, quoted in Hurd-Mead, *History of Women*, 143.

## Hildegard of Bingen

1 E. Petroff, *Medieval Women's Visionary Literature*, 6.

2 Lynn Thorndike, *A History of Magic and Experimental Science*, vol. 2, 126.

3 Ibid, 128.

4 See Wighard Strehlow and Gottfried Hertzka, *Hildegard of Bingen's Medicine*, trans. Karl Kaiser, xx.

5 Ibid, ixx.

6 Ibid, xx.

7 Dronke, trans., *Women Writers of the Middle Ages*, 180–81.

8 See Barbara Newman, *Sister of Wisdom: St Hildegard's Theology of the Feminine*, 118.

9 Dronke, *Women Writers*, 175.

10 Newman, *Sister of Wisdom*, 130.

11 Ibid, 135.

12 Ibid, 141.

13 Dronke, *Women Writers*, 178; see also ibid, 141–42.

14 Thorndike, *History of Magic*, 150.

15 Ibid, 151.

16 Dronke, *Women Writers*, 178.

17 Newman, *Sister of Wisdom*, 145.

18 Ibid, 148.

19 Fiona Bowie and Oliver Davies, quoting Dronke in *Hildegard of Bingen: An Anthology*, 32.

20 Sabina Flanagan, *Hildegard of Bingen*, 83.

21 Ibid, 86.

22 Thorndike, *History of Magic*, 140.

23 Flanagan, *Hildegard*, 95.

24 Thorndike, *History of Magic*, 154.

25 *Liber Vitae Meritorum*, Book II. (Hildegard's medicine.) See Strehlow and Hertzka, *Hildegard*, 133.

## Women Physicians in the Late Middle Ages

1 Jeanne Achterburg, *Woman as Healer*, 77.

2 Ibid.

3 Kate Campbell Hurd-Mead, "Concerning Certain Medical Women of the Late Middle Ages," *Medical Life,* XLII (January–December 1935): 114.

4 Anna Comnena, *The Alexiad,* book 2, section 10, Elizabeth Davies, trans., In Muriel Hughes, *Women Healers in Medieval Life and Literature,* 37–38.

5 Margaret Alic, *Hypatia's Heritage,* 47–48.

6 Ibid, 48.

7 Hurd-Mead, "Concerning Certain Medical Women," 115.

8 Charter of the University of Paris, II, 257–68, quoted in Hillary Bourdillon, *Women as Healers,* 15.

9 Charter of the University of Paris, II, 263–65, quoted in Pearl Kibre, "The Faculty of Medicine at Paris," *Bulletin of the History of Medicine,* XXVII (1953).

10 Charter of the University of Paris, II, 257–58, quoted in Bourdillon, *Women as Healers,* 15.

11 Hughes, *Women Healers,* 42.

## The Struggle to Practice: Women Healers Under Threat

1 Matilda Gage, *Women, Church and State,* 105.

2 Ibid, quoting Mitchelet, *La Sorciere,* note 36 to chapter 5, 272.

3 Ibid, 102.

4 Ibid, 105.

5 See Penelope Shuttle and Peter Redgrove, *The Wise Wound.*

6 Susan Griffin, *Woman and Nature,* 95.

7 The Bible, Book of Revelation, quoted in Anthony Wilson, *The Female Pest,* 7.

8 Mary Daly, *Gyn/Ecology,* 183.

9 Jeanne Achterberg, *Woman as Healer,* 90.

10 Montague Summers, *Malleus Maleficarum,* Part I, Q II, 66.

11 Quoted in Sophia Jex-Blake, *Medical Women,* 16.

12 Ibid.

13 Ibid, 16–17.

14 Ibid, 17.

15 Barbara Ehrenreich and Deirdre English, *Witches, Midwives and Nurses,* 15.

16 Keith Thomas, *Religion and the Decline of Magic,* 14.

17 Ibid.

18 Summers, *Malleus Maleficarum,* 220.

19 Mary Daly, *Gyn/Ecology,* 194.

20 Gage, *Women, Church,* 100.

21 J. B. Russell, *Witchcraft in the Middle Ages,* 266.

22 Ibid, 282.

23 Gillian Tindall, *A Handbook on Witches,* 34.

24 Ibid, 148.

25 Daly, *Gyn/Ecology,* 202.

26 Walker, *Woman's Encyclopaedia,* 445.

27 See G. G. Coulton, *Life in the Middle Ages,* vol. 1, *Religion, Folk-Lore and Superstition,* 32.

28 Russell, *Witchcraft,* 276, discussing J. Glenn Gray's *The Warriors,* 26.

29 Ibid.

30 Charles Hoyt, *Witchcraft,* 96.

31 Gregory Zilboorg, *The Medical Man and the Witch During the Renaissance,* 26.

32 Ibid, 66–70.

33 Ibid, 69–70.

34 Christina Larner, *Enemies of God: The Witchhunt in Scotland,* 89–102.

35 Ibid, 96.

36 Norman Cohn, *Europe's Inner Demons,* 258–59.

37 Montague Summers, *The History of Witchcraft and Demonology,* xiv.

38 Ian Maclean, *The Renaissance Notion of Women,* 2.

39 Ibid, 8, 36.

40 Ibid, 36.

41 Ibid, 41.

42 Ibid, 85.

43 Ibid, 46.

# Women Healers from the Sixteenth to the Eighteenth Century

1 Alice Clark, *Working Life of Women in the Seventeenth Century,* 258.

2 Ibid.

3 Ibid, 259.

4 Sarah Fell, *Household Accounts,* 95, in Clark, ibid, 255.

5 *The Life and Death of Lady Lettice Falkland,* in Clark, ibid, 256.

6 *The Life and Death of William Bedell,* 2, in Clark, ibid.

7 R. Josselin, *Diary,* 1672, 163–64, in Clark, ibid, 257.

8 *The Life of Marmaduke Rawdon,* 85, in Clark, ibid.

9 See Hurd-Mead, *History of Women,* 352–53.

10 Jane Sharp, *The Midwives Book or the Whole Art of Midwifery Discovered,* first edition 1671; *The Compleat Midwives Companion,* fourth edition, 1725, in Clark, *Working Life,* 270–71.

11 From Nicholas Culpeper, *Directory for Midwives*, in Clark, ibid, 271–72.

12 *A Scheme for Foundation of a Royal Hospital, Harleian Miscellany*, vol. IV, 142–47, in Clark, ibid, 273.

13 See Hurd-Mead, *History of Women*, 401.

14 The work was entitled *Observations diverses sur la stérilite, perte de fruiet, fécondite achouchements et maladies des femmes et des enfants nouveaux naiz; amplement traites et heureusement practiquees par Loyse Bourgeois, dite Bousier, sage-femme de la Royne.*

15 See Hurd-Mead, *History of Women*, 411.

16 Ibid, 425.

17 See Melina Lipinska, *Histoire des femmes medicins depuis L'antiquite jusqu'a nos jours,* 78.

18 Hurd-Mead, *History of Women*, 431.

19 Margaret Nicholas, *The World's Wickedest Women,* (London; Octopus Books, 1984) 103–9.

20 See Hurd-Mead, *History of Women*, 432–33.

21 Letters of the Right Honorable Lady Montague, April 1917, vol 1, 84–85. See Hurd-Mead, *History of Women*, 469 and Alic, *Hypatia's Heritage*, 89.

22 Ibid.

# Women Enter the Profession: The Struggles of Nineteenth-Century Women Doctors

1 Elizabeth Blackwell, *Pioneer Work in Opening the Medical Profession to Women,* 190.

2 Mary Roth Walsh, "Doctors wanted: No Women Need Apply," *Sexual Barriers in the Medical Profession 1835–1975,* 2.

3 See Jeanne Achterberg, *Woman as Healer,* 142.

4 Walsh, *"Doctors Wanted,"* 30.

5 Ibid.

6 Quoted in Achterberg, *Woman as Healer,* 143.

7 Elizabeth Blackwell, quoted in Catriona Blake, *The Charge of the Parasols,* 31.

8 Blackwell, *Pioneer Work,* 60–61.

9 Ibid, 62.

10 Ibid, 70.

11 Ibid. Quoted in Blake, *The Charge,* 32.

12 Blackwell, *Pioneer Work,* 197–98.

13 Ibid, 141.

14 See Daly, *Gyn/Ecology,* 225.

15 Ibid, 228.

16 G. J. Barker-Benfield, *Horrors of a Half Known Life: Male Attitudes Toward Women and Sexuality in Nineteenth-century America*, 83.

17 Ely Van de Warker, "The Fetich of the Ovary," *American Journal of Obstetrics* 54, no. 3, (September 1906): 371.

18 A. Vietor, *A Woman's Quest: The Life of Marie E. Zakrzewska, MD*, 84–85.

19 The *Lancet*, 6 July 1861, 16.

20 Quoted in Blake, *The Charge*, 67–68.

21 Ibid, 68.

22 Jex-Blake, *Medical Women*, 53.

23 Ibid, 96.

24 *The English Woman's Review* (January 1870): 28.

25 See Jex-Blake's comments on the decision in *Medical Women*, 59.

26 Robert Wilson writing to Edith Pechey, 20 November 1870, quoted in Margaret Todd, *The Life of Sophia Jex-Blake*, 294.

27 *British Medical Journal* 1 (20 January, 1912).

28 Jex-Blake, *Medical Women*, 161.

29 Mary Seacole, *The Wonderful Adventures of Mrs Seacole in Many Lands*, 56.

30 Ibid, 76.

31 Ibid, 78.

32 Ibid, 83.

33 Ibid, 125.

34 Ibid, 127.

35 Ibid, 145–46.

36 Ibid, 195.

37 *The Times*, Editorial, 11 April, 1857, quoted in ibid, 208.

## Persecution Through Committee

1 Wendy Savage, *A Savage Enquiry*, 59.

2 Senior obstetrician, quoted in the *Sunday Times*, 9 March 1986, in Savage, *Savage Enquiry*, xv.

3 "Correspondence," *British Medical Journal*, 297 (29 October 1985): 1125.

4 Soo Downe, "Blind Justice," *Nursing Times* 85, no. 5, (1 February 1989): 24.

5 *British Medical Journal* 297 (29 October 1988): 1125.

6 Ibid.

7 Justice Watkins, "The Case of Rosser vs UK Central Council for Nursing, Midwifery and Health Visiting," *Nursing Times* 85, no. 12 (22 March 1989): 19.

8 Caroline Flint, "A Matter of Judgement," *Nursing Times*, ibid, 19.

9 *British Medical Journal,* 297 (29 October 1988): 811.

10 Caroline Sadler, "Going it Alone," *Nursing Times* 84, no. 23 (8 June 1988): 16.

11 Savage, *Savage Enquiry,* xvi.

12 Ibid.

13 Ibid, 5.

14 Ibid, 16.

15 Ibid, 22.

16 Ibid, 23.

17 Ibid, xvi.

18 Ibid, 175.

19 Ibid, 176.

20 Ibid, 177.

21 Michael O'Donnell, *British Medical Journal* (May 1986), quoted in ibid, 72.

22 Savage, *Savage Enquiry,* 74.

23 Ibid, 119.

24 Ibid, 163.

25 "Lessons from the Savage Enquiry," *British Medical Journal* 293 (2 August 1986): 285.

26 Ibid, 286.

27 *Daily Telegraph,* 12 July 1986, quoted in Savage, *Savage Enquiry,* 173.

28 "Professional implications of the Savage Case," *Lancet* (12 April 1986): 837.

29 See Beatrix Campbell, *Unofficial Secrets.*

30 Ibid, 4–5.

31 lbid, 73.

32 Ibid.

33 Ibid, 5.

34 Ibid, 50.

35 Ibid, 53.

36 Ibid, 61.

37 Ibid, 86.

38 Ibid.

39 Ibid, 95.

40 Harvey Marcovitch, "The Media on the Cleveland Affair," *British Medical Journal* 297 (16 July 1988): 233.

# Women Shamans and Conjurers

1 For menstruation as a polluting force, see Penelope Shuttle and Peter Redgrove, *The Wise Wound.*

2 Vicki Noble, *Motherpeace*, 76.

3 Erich Neumann, *The Great Mother*, 294–97.

4 Ibid, 295.

5 Noble, *Motherpeace*, 108.

6 See Frank Jerome, *Persuasion and Healing*, 285–89.

7 Susan Griffin, *Women and Nature*, 1.

8 Bobette Perrone, H. Henrietta Stockel, and Victoria Krueger, *Medicine Women, Curanderas and Women Doctors*, 22.

9 See Gray, "Rediscovering Native American Medicine," *East West Journal* (November, 1986): 15.

10 Hartley Burr Alexander, *The Mythology of All Races*, vol. 10, *North American*, 1916, 91.

11 Ibid, 91.

12 Ibid, 92.

13 See Merlin Stone, "Pasowee, the Buffalo Woman," in *Ancient Mirrors of Womanhood*, 307–8.

14 Perrone, Stockel and Krueger, *Medicine Women*, 33.

15 Ibid, 36.

16 Ibid, 38.

17 Ibid, 40.

18 Ibid, 41.

19 Information drawn from Barbara Kerewsky-Halpem, "Serbian Conjurers' Word Magic," in *Women as Healers: Cross-Cultural Perspectives*, Carol Shepherd, ed.

20 Ibid, 127.

21 Ibid.

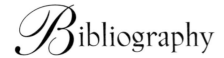

# Bibliography

Achterberg, Jeanne. *Woman as Healer.* London: Rider, 1990.

Alexander, Hartley Burr. *The Mythology of All Races.* Vol. 10, *North American.* Boston: Marshall Jones Co. 1916.

Alic, Margaret. *Hypatia's Heritage: A History of Women in Science from Antiquity to the late Nineteenth Century.* London: The Women's Press, 1986.

Barker-Benfield, G. J. *Horrors of a Half Known Life: Male Attitudes Towards Women and Sexuality in Nineteenth-century America.* New York: Harper & Row, 1976.

Blackwell, Elizabeth. *Pioneer Work in Opening the Medical Profession to Women.* London: Longmans, Green and Co., 1895.

Blake, Catriona. *The Charge of the Parasols: Women's Entry to the Medical Profession.* London: The Women's Press, 1990.

Bourdillon, Hillary. *Women as Healers: A History of Women and Medicine.* Cambridge: Cambridge University Press, 1988.

Bowie, Fiona, and Oliver Davies. *Hildegard of Bingen: An Anthology.* London: SPCK, 1990.

Bradley, Marion. *The Mists of Avalon.* London: Michael Joseph, 1983.

Brooke, Elisabeth. *A Woman's Book of Herbs.* London: The Women's Press, 1992.

Bryan, Cyril P., trans. *The Papyrus Ebers.* London: Geoffrey Bles, 1929.

Campbell, Beatrix. *Unofficial Secrets: Child Sexual Abuse—The Cleveland Case.* London: Virago, 1989.

Clark, Alice. *Working Life of Women in the Seventeenth Century.* London: George Routledge & Sons, 1919.

Cohn, Norman. *Europe's Inner Demons: an enquiry inspired by the great witch-hunt.* London: Sussex University Press, 1975.

Coulton, G. G. *Life in the Middle Ages. Vol. 1, Religion, Folk-Lore and Superstition.* Cambridge: Cambridge University Press, 1910.

Culpeper, Nicholas. *Culpeper's Complete Herbal and English Physician.* Manchester: J. Gleave and Son, Deansgate, 1826.

Daly, Mary. *Gyn/Ecology: The Metaethics of Radical Feminism.* London: The Women's Press, 1979.

Dronke, Peter. *Women Writers of the Middle Ages.* Cambridge: Cambridge University Press, 1984.

Ehrenreich, Barbara, and Deirdre English. *Witches, Midwives and Nurses.* Old Westbury: Feminist Press, New York, 1974.

Flanagan, Sabina. *Hildegard of Bingen, 1098–1179: A Visionary Life.* London: Routledge, 1989.

Gage, Matilda Joslyn. *Women, Church and State.* 1893. Reprint. Watertown, Mass.: Persephone Press, 1980.

Griffin, Susan. *Woman and Nature: The Roaring Inside Her.* London: The Women's Press, 1984.

Griffith, F. L., ed. *The Petrie Papyri, Hieratic Papyri from Kahun and Gurob.* London: Bernard Quaritch, 1898.

Hoyt, Charles Alva. *Witchcraft.* Carbondale and Edwardsville: Southern Illinois University Press 1981.

Hughes, Muriel Joy. *Women Healers in Medieval Life and Literature.* New York: King's Crown Press, 1943.

Hurd-Mead, Kate Campbell. *A History of Women in Medicine: from the earliest times to the beginning of the nineteenth century.* Haddam, Conn.: The Haddam Press, 1938.

Jerome, Frank. *Persuasion and Healing: A Comparative Study of Psychotherapy.* New York: Johns Hopkins University Press, 1974.

Jex-Blake, Sophia. *Medical Women.* Edinburgh: Oliphant, Anderson and Ferrier, 1886.

Larner, Christina. *Enemies of God: The Witchhunt in Scotland.* London: Chatto & Windus, 1981.

Leake, Chauncey D. *The Old Egyptian Medical Papyri.* Lawrence, Kansas: University of Kansas Press, 1952.

Lipinska, Melina. *Histoire des femmes medicins depuis L'antiquite jusqu'a nos jours.* Paris: G. Jaques & Co., 1930.

McKenzie, Dan. *The Infancy of Medicine.* London: Macmillan, 1925.

Maclean, Ian. *The Renaissance Notion of Woman.* Cambridge: Cambridge University Press, 1980. Manton, Jo. *Elizabeth Garrett-Anderson.* London: A. and C. Black, 1958.

Mason-Hohl, Elizabeth, trans. *The Diseases of Women by Trotula of Salerno: a translation of Passioni-bus Mulierum Curandorum.* Hollywood, Calif.: The Ward Ritchie Press, 1940.

Mozans, H. J. *Women in Science.* New York and London: D. Appleton and Co., 1913.

Newman, Barbara. *Sister of Wisdom: St Hildegard's Theology of the Feminine.* Berkeley and Los Angeles: University of California Press, 1987.

Neumann, Erich. *The Great Mother: An Analysis of the Archetype.* Princeton, New Jersey: Routledge & Kegan Paul, 1972. [First published 1963.]

Noble, Vicki. *Motherpeace: A Way to the Goddess through Myth, Art and Tarot.* San Francisco: Harper & Row, 1985.

Pagels, Elaine. *The Gnostic Gospels.* New York: Random House, 1979.

Perrone, Bobette, H. Henrietta Stockel, and Victoria Krueger. *Medicine Women, Curanderas and Women Doctors.* Oklahoma: University of Oklahoma Press, 1989.

Petroff, E. *Medieval Women's Visionary Literature.* Oxford: Oxford University Press, 1986.

Rhode, Eleanour Sinclair. *The Old English Herbals.* London: Longmans, Green and Co., 1922.

Robbins, Rossell Hope. Th*e Encyclopedia of Witchcraft and Demonology.* London: Spring Books, 1959.

Russell, Jeffrey Barton. W*itchcraft in the Middle Ages.* Ithaca and London: Cornell University Press, 1972.

Savage, Wendy. *A Savage Enquiry: Who Controls Childbirth?* London: Virago, 1986.

Seacole, Mary. *The Wonderful Adventures of Mrs Seacole in Many Lands.* 1857. Reprint. London: James Blackwood, 1984.

Shepherd, Carol, ed. *Women as Healers: Cross-Cultural Perspectives.* London: Rutgers, 1989.

Shuttle, Penelope and Redgrove, Peter. *The Wise Wound.* London: Penguin, 1978.

Stone, Merlin. *Ancient Mirrors of Womanhood.* Boston: Beacon Press, 1979.

Strehlow, Wighard, and Gottfried Hertzka. *Hildegard of Bingen's Medicine.* Santa Fe, New Mexico: Bear & Co, 1988.

Summers, Montague. *The History of Witchcraft and Demonology.* London: Kegan Paul, 1926.

————trans. *Malleus Maleficarum,* London: The Pushkin Press, 1948. [First edition 1928.]

Thomas, Keith. *Religion and the Decline of Magic: Studies in Popular Beliefs in Sixteenth and Seventeenth-century England.* London: Weidenfeld and Nicolson, 1971.

Thompson, R. C. *Assyrian Medical Texts, from the originals in the British Museum.* Oxford: Oxford University Press, 1924.

Thorndike, Lynn. A History of Magic and Experimental Science. 8 vols. New York: Columbia University Press, 1923–1958.

Tindall, Gillian. A *Handbook on Witches.* London: Arthur Barker, 1965.

Todd, Margaret. *The Life of Sophia Jex-Blake.* London: Macmillan, 1918.

Vietor, A. *A Woman's Quest: The Life of Marie E. Zakrzewska, MD.* New York and London: D. Appleton and Co., 1924.

Walker, Barbara. *The Woman's Encyclopaedia of Myths and Secrets.* San Francisco: Harper & Row, 1983.

Walsh, Mary Roth. "Doctors Wanted, No Women Need Apply" in *Sexual Barriers in the Medical Profession 1835–1975.* New Haven: Yale University Press, 1977.

Wilson, Anthony. *The Female Pest: an exposé of misogynist mythology.* London: Anthony Wilson, 1985.

Zilboorg, Gregory. *The Medical Man and the Witch During the Renaissance.* Baltimore: The Johns Hopkins Press, 1935.

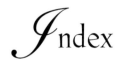

# Index